USMLE STEP 2 CS FOR THE IMG

The Ultimate Review Guidebook for the International Medical Graduate

Victor S. Flauta, M.D.

USMLE STEP 2 CS FOR THE IMG

The Ultimate Review Guidebook for the International Medical Graduate

Victor S. Flauta, M.D.
Pathology Resident
University of Missouri-Kansas City
Truman Medical Centers
Kansas City, Missouri

To the helpless victims

of the December 2004 earthquake and tsunami

that claimed

the lives of thousands and

broke the hearts of millions

Cover and book design: 1106 Design, LLC
Copyediting: Kate von Seeburg
Index preparation: Doran Hunter

ISBN 0-7414-2626-9

Published by:

INFINITY PUBLISHING.COM

1094 New De Haven Street, Suite 100
West Conshohocken, PA 19428-2713
Info@buybooksontheweb.com
www.buybooksontheweb.com
Toll-free (877) BUY BOOK
Local Phone (610) 941-9999
Fax (610) 941-9959

Printed in the United States of America

Printed on Recycled Paper

Published June 2005

A portion of the proceeds

from the sale of this book

will be donated to

rebuilding efforts in South Asia.

INTRODUCTION AND ACKNOWLEDGMENT

This book was created out of necessity. When I was reviewing for the clinical skills exam, I scoured the Internet for a review book that deals with this subject matter. At that time, my options were very limited. I needed a book that would address the issues confronting IMGs when they take this exam — a review book that would tell me how to pose questions and offer explanations during the interview process and how to do things properly during the physical examination. When I couldn't find one, I started making my own. I never expected this to become a book, but as I went through my review, a few sheets of paper with scribbled notes were transformed into useful sheets I found very valuable when I took the exam.

This book is divided into two parts. The first section deals with an easy-to-follow Frequently Asked Questions (FAQs). Here, I attempted to provide the answers to questions a Step 2 CS candidate might have. The second section is a collection of sample patient encounters on cases that are commonly seen in a typical U.S. clinic or hospital. IMG physicians will find this book more useful if they practice these mock encounters with a study partner to reinforce the learning and familiarity process. By doing so, they will be able to manage their time more efficiently, which is a crucial factor in establishing confidence for the actual exam.

Like any publication, this undertaking is a collaborative enterprise which would not have come into fruition without the help of various individuals and institutions. I would like to express my gratitude to Dr. Yuen Qian who had been my study partner during our mock encounters. His clinical insights, valuable suggestions and constructive criticisms have been indispensable in the creation of this book. Special thanks are also due to several IMG physicians who have peer-reviewed the manuscript. Their corrections and recommendations have made this guide book a much better one. I also feel obligated to thank Yale University School of Medicine for giving me the privilege of a cardiology clerkship and the Texas Scottish Rite Hospital for Children in Dallas for an observership in pediatrics orthopedics. Both experiences provided me a ringside view of the U.S. healthcare system which have become the foundation for a lot of the practical and clinical opinions expressed in this book. My indebtedness extends to my family in the Philippines for their unparalleled intellectual and emotional support. I also want to thank my wife, Lynette, for her patience and continuous support of my medical and journalistic endeavors. And to my sons, Brandon and Matthew, who kept stepping and punching unwanted characters on my laptop while I worked on this project. Their toddler pranks were nothing compared to the inspiration they provide me everyday.

Finally, I hope that the readers will provide feedback, in order that subsequent editions will become an improved version of its predecessor. Please e-mail all comments to *step2cs@sbcglobal.net.*

—Victor S. Flauta, M.D.

TABLE OF CONTENTS

Part II: Mock Exam

Part I:
FAQ

Chapter 1

An Introduction to the USMLE Step 2 CS

"Best decisions are informed decisions."
— Anonymous

- **What is the Step 2 CS?**
- **Who can take Step 2 CS?**
- **What is the difference between the Step 2 CS (Step 2 CS) and the Clinical Skills Assessment (CSA)?**
- **I have already passed the CSA. Do I still have to take the Step 2 CS?**
- **What are the prerequisites to taking the Step 2 CS?**
- **How often is the Step 2 CS administered?**
- **Where is it administered?**
- **How much is the application fee?**
- **Whom do I contact for information regarding the Step 2 CS?**
- **How do I schedule my exam?**
- **There are two sessions available — a morning (AM) and an afternoon (PM) session. Can I choose between the two sessions?**
- **What clinical disciplines are covered in the Step 2 CS?**
- **How long is the Step 2 CS certification valid?**

GENERAL INFORMATION

What is the Step 2 CS?

USMLE Step 2 consists of two parts: Step 2 Clinical Knowledge (Step 2 CK) and the Step 2 Clinical Skills (Step 2 CS). Step 2 CK determines the examinee's theoretical knowledge of medicine while Step 2 CS gauges his data gathering, physical examination and communication skills. Completion of USMLE Step 2 requires passage of both these two components.

Who can take Step 2 CS?

Medical students, graduates of U.S. and Canadian medical schools, and International Medical Graduates (IMGs) can take this test.

What is the difference between the Step 2 CS (Step 2 CS) and the Clinical Skills Assessment (CSA)?

Clinical Skills Assessment (CSA) was the immediate precursor to the Step 2 CS, and it used to be administered by the Educational Commission for Foreign Medical Graduate (ECFMG) to international medical graduates as a requirement for ECFMG certification. It is no longer administered since it has been replaced by the Step 2 CS. CSA had an expiration of three years after passage while Step 2 CS does not expire once it is passed. Other differences are tabulated in the USMLE website.

I have already passed the CSA. Do I still have to take the Step 2 CS?

No. According to the USMLE official website, those who have passed the previously administered CSA do not have to take the Step 2 CS.

ELIGIBILITY

What are the prerequisites to taking the Step 2 CS?

Applicants must have passed the USMLE Step 1 to be eligible to take this exam. U.S. and Canadian medical students must be officially enrolled in a medical school in the U.S. or Canada, while IMGs must be officially enrolled or must have graduated from a medical school listed in the International Medical Education Directory (IMED).

TEST DATES

How often is the Step 2 CS administered?

It is offered regularly throughout the year.

LOCATION

Where is it administered?

There are five clinical skills evaluation centers in the United States: which include Atlanta, Chicago, Houston, Los Angeles and Philadelphia. Their addresses are printed below. It is presently not being administered outside the United States.

1. Clinical Skills Evaluation Center — Atlanta
   Two Crown Center
   1745 Phoenix Boulevard, Suite 500
   Atlanta, GA 30349

2. Clinical Skills Evaluation Center — Chicago
   Crossroads Center at O'Hare
   6th Floor
   8501 West Higgins Rd.
   Chicago, IL 60631

3. Clinical Skills Evaluation Center — Houston
   400 North Sam Houston Parkway, Suite 700
   Houston, TX 77060

4. Clinical Skills Evaluation Center — Los Angeles
   Pacific Corporate Towers
   13th Floor
   100 North Sepulveda Boulevard
   El Segundo, CA 90245

5. Clinical Skills Evaluation Center — Philadelphia
   3624 Market Street, 3rd Floor
   Philadelphia, PA 19104

How much is the application fee?

$1,200. Ouch! So make sure you pass it the first time.

Whom do I contact for information regarding the Step 2 CS?

If you are an IMG contact:
ECFMG
3624 Market St. Philadelphia, PA 19104-2685, USA
Telephone: (215) 386-5900 Fax: (215) 386-9196
Website: http://www.ecfmg.org
E-mail: info@ecfmg.org

If you are a U.S. or Canadian medical student contact:
NBME Examinee Support Services
3750 Market Street Philadelphia, PA 19104-3190
Telephone: (215) 590-9700 Fax: (215) 590-9457
Website: http://www.nbme.org
E-mail: webmail@nbme.org

SCHEDULING

How do I schedule my exam?

There are two ways to do this. The first and easiest is through the Internet. Go to *http://www.ecfmg.org* and click on Step 2 CS. You will only be able to enter the Step 2 CS scheduling page if you are registered for the exam. Once you're in it, you can choose the year, month and day for your exam. You can also schedule by calling the ECFMG/Step 2 CS office at (215) 970-1982. The office is open Monday through Friday from 8 a.m. to 5 p.m., Eastern Standard Time.

There are different time zones in the United States — the Pacific, Mountain, Central and Eastern Time zones. Because the exam is administered in five different locations in the U.S., you have to consider these four different time zones when you schedule your exam. Philadelphia, Chicago and Atlanta follow the Eastern Standard Time zone; Houston follows the Central Time zone; and Los Angeles follows the Pacific Time zone.

Several sites on the Internet let you find out what time it is in any major city in the world. Just type "time zones" in yahoo.com or google.com and you can pick from a list of options. Considering the enormous long distance charges you are likely to incur if you call, scheduling your exam via the Internet is less expensive and more efficient. After you receive your permit, you must schedule your exam as soon as possible. If you reschedule your exam date with more than 30 days advance notice, you will pay a rescheduling fee of $50. As of this writing, this fee is being indefinitely waived. However, if you reschedule your exam within 30 days of your exam date, you will pay a rescheduling fee of $150.

There are two sessions available — a morning (AM) and an afternoon (PM) session. Can I choose between the two sessions?

No. You will be assigned either the morning or afternoon session and are not given a choice.

CLINICAL DISCIPLINES

What clinical disciplines are covered in the Step 2 CS?

The ECFMG bulletin states that the exam can cover cases from internal medicine, family medicine, OB-GYN, surgery, pediatrics, psychiatry including each field's subspecialty areas. In other words, anything under the sun. But these are usually the most common cases you will see in a typical U.S. clinic, hospital or emergency room. These cases are not distributed equally from among the major areas so it is possible, for example, to be faced with nine cases from internal medicine and two cases from psychiatry or — three from internal medicine, two from family medicine, two from obstetrics and gynecology, two from surgery and two from psychiatry. Be prepared to encounter a variety of cases and practice mock encounters for each discipline.

How long is the Step 2 CS certification valid?

It has no expiration date so, basically, it is valid forever. The previous CSA was valid for three years. If you did not obtain a residency position within that time frame, you would have to take the exam again.

Chapter 2

Preparing for the Examination

"Half-baked results are often due to half-baked commitments."
—V. S. Flauta

- **What is the best time to take the Step 2 CS?**
- **How long should I review for the exam?**
- **What do you suggest taking first, the USMLE Step 2 CK or the USMLE Step 2 CS?**
- **What is the best way to prepare?**
- **Where can I contact other people who might be interested in becoming a study partner?**
- **What review books should I buy?**
- **How about review courses?**
- **Are there any available tutorial DVDs or CDs available?**
- **What should I do to get some actual clinical experience in the United States?**
- **Where can I get a list of institutions that offer observerships?**
- **Do residency programs offer observerships?**
- **Are institutions with residency programs my only choice for observership?**

TIME

What is the best time to take the Step 2 CS?

You have many things to consider when deciding on the best day for the Step 2 CS. Usually, interviews for the residency training start in November (some institutions start interviewing in September) and end in January or February, depending on the program. That means you should have your Step 2 CS result before November. Because it takes about six to eight weeks before ECFMG releases your Step 2 CS result, you can schedule your exam anytime from April to August.

And while waiting for the result, you can register with ERAS (Electronic Residency Application Service) and start working on your documents. Make sure that you select an option in ERAS where your USMLE transcript will be automatically updated with the results of your other tests. This will save you time later on, and it's one less hassle in your agenda. After the November to February interview period, the "moment of truth" arrives in March and you'll find out if you were matched or not. If you aren't matched, you may have to stay a little longer in the U.S. for the post-match, to try your luck in the much-dreaded scramble. You only have three months to work on this because almost all programs start in July. In reality, you only have a few days to see if lady luck is on your side, because those vacant slots fill up quickly. In summary, you have to schedule your Step 2 CS based on this timetable.

How long should I review for the exam?

If you have not seen a clinical patient for quite a while, you may need a few to several months of brushing up on your clinical knowledge and skills. If you recently graduated, I believe a few weeks of practice with a study partner should suffice.

What do you suggest taking first, the USMLE Step 2 CK or the USMLE Step 2 CS?

I'd take Step 2 CK first before I take the Step 2 CS. Your Step 2 CK review will boost your confidence in Step 2 CS because you will find it easier to make a differential diagnosis and relevant work-ups since you've recently gone through them during your review for the Step 2 CK. Taking the Step 2 CS first won't help you pass the Step 2 CK and may even pull you down if you do not put enough time between them.

Another factor is that the Step 2 CS is more difficult to schedule than the Step 2 CK, because the CK portion is administered in many Sylvan Prometric branches around the world, while the CS portion is only administered in five locations in the U.S. Thus, getting the CK out of the way will help you with better scheduling.

Third, some program directors will give an interview if you have passed both Step 1 and Step 2 CK, even if your Step 2 CS is pending. You will rarely find a program that will give you an interview if you have not yet passed the CK portion of the exam.

Fourth, because the percentage of IMGs failing the CK portion for the first time is significantly higher than those failing the CS part, it is better to pass the CK portion first. Once it is passed, the likelihood of passing the CS portion is much greater. On the other hand, passing the CS does not increase the likelihood of passing the CK. I wouldn't risk my $1,200 (plus hotel, airline and car rental fees) until after I am through with the CK portion.

My suggested strategy is to take these tests accordingly: Step 1, Step 2 CK, Step 2 CS, and TOEFL. I'd take the TOEFL last because it is only good for two years. You may end up taking it again if you do not pass any of the other tests within the two-year period so take it last and save yourself some money.

STUDY PARTNER

What is the best way to prepare?

I think the best preparation for the Step 2 CS is a mock encounter with a study partner. You can act as a doctor and your partner can act as the standardized patient, then switch places. The advantage of this strategy is the interaction — the sharing of ideas, the challenging questions you both will throw at each other, and the confidence you will build after you have done several mock encounters. Most importantly, it is very affordable because it is free! There are other review materials available, but nothing replaces the actual practice encounters a study partner can provide. There are also review classes for Step 2 CS offered by Kaplan, including a one-day course and a five-day course. The one-day course won't be sufficient if you haven't seen a clinical patient for a long time. The five-day course is probably the best if you have the time and money. The only advantage I see with these Kaplan courses is the simulation of the real Step 2 CS. Considering all factors, I think the best way to prepare is the mock encounters with a study partner for one to two months plus a one-day Kaplan Step 2 CS simulation.

Where can I contact other people who might be interested in becoming a study partner?

Go online, join one of the forums, and post a note that you are seeking a study partner in your particular city. Leave an e-mail address or a telephone number so they can contact you. You might find the following online sites useful:

1. Prep4usmle.com
2. Usmle.net
3. ValueMD.com
4. Network 54
5. PinoyImg

Go to Google or Yahoo and type "USMLE forum" and you will see other sites that offer similar discussion groups.

REVIEW BOOKS

What review books should I buy?

Don't buy. Borrow, instead. If you feel more comfortable owning your resource materials, look for the following available books:

Mastering the Objective Structured Clinical Examination and the Clinical Skills Assessment by Jo-Ann Reteguiz, Beverly Cornel-Avendano *$39.95*
Presents more than 60 standardized patient practice cases, focuses on the interviewing and physical exam skills, and provides key history-taking and physical exam pearls. (This book is a good reference to have for Step 2 CS.)

First Aid for the USMLE Step 2 CS by Vikas Bhushan, Tao Le *$34.95*
Another book from the First Aid series featuring frequently tested cases, strategies for challenging patient encounters and good discussions on about 27+ completely simulated cases. (I highly recommend this book.)

NMS Review for the Clinical Skills Assessment Exam by Erich A. Arias *$36.95*
This book was created as a review material for the Clinical Skills Assessment (Step 2 CS) exam which is now replaced by the USMLE Step 2 CS. Features examples, figures and tables, and a review of clinical exam and medical history in a variety of disciplines. (Good reading but not as useful as the first two books listed.)

Bates' Guide to Physical Examination & History Taking (Book + CD-ROM) by Lynn S. Bickley, Peter G. Szilagyi *$72.95*
This material provides a foundation for learning physical examination and history taking with emphasis on procedures, interpretations, and common abnormalities. Numerous color and halftone illustrations are included. (Excellent for medical school but not the best for Step 2 CS; borrow if you can.)

Textbook of Physical Diagnosis: History and Examination with CD-ROM by Mark H. Swartz *$72.95*
This new edition was updated to reflect the most current standards of physical diagnosis. New color images replace many old black-and-white images, and more than 200 new color photographs of pathological conditions make this edition a lot better than the previous one. Includes a free CD-ROM featuring a video demonstration of the complete physical examination of a man and the breast and pelvic examinations of a woman. (Very good reference but a little pricey because it is hard bound. Buy this one if you can afford it. You will find the CD that comes with it very helpful.)

Lecture Notes on Clinical Skills by Roger Blackwood, Chris Hatton *$41.95*
Pocket-sized outline for medical students and residents. Covers essential principles and techniques of history taking and examination, and provides guidance on the key professional skills involved in developing and maintaining good communication between doctor and patient. (Borrow if you can.)

Pocket Companion for Textbook of Physical Diagnosis by Mark H. Swartz *$41.97*
This is the "baby" version of Dr. Swartz's *Textbook of Physical Diagnosis: History and Examination, 3rd Edition.* Concise, user-friendly and very useful for residents and clinicians but may not be as good for Step 2 CS. (I'd rather buy the "mother" version of this book for an additional $30 which includes a CD-ROM.)

CS Checklists: Portable Review for the USMLE Step 2 CS by Jennifer K. Rooney *$29.95*
Features 45 frequently-tested CS cases including their typical presentations, history, physical exams, and differential diagnosis. Points out the most essential clinical knowledge and skills you will need in the clinic — and on the Step 2 CS exam.

Kaplan Medical USMLE Step 2 Clinical Skills by Kaplan Medical *$34.95*
Prepared by Kaplan, this book guides readers through this challenging, standardized patient exam. It includes advice and information about the following topics: clinical reasoning, doctor-patient communication, performing a focused history and physical exam, writing the patient note, establishing a differential diagnosis and, how to avoid the common mistakes that can impact exam performance.

I think the best material out there is probably the Kaplan review notes, but you will only get this if you enroll in their five-day course. If you can borrow one from a friend, well and good — but don't photocopy them because of copyright infringement issues. Some are offering these notes in some of the online forums but be sure you don't thread upon illegal waters. Make sure they are legitimate original copies and make sure you aren't dealing with a sleazy con artist.

In summary, the aforementioned publications are valuable medical resources, but choose and buy only one additional book (alongside the one you are holding right now) to reinforce your knowledge and confidence for the exam. Buying more than two books will create redundancy and confusion. In my opinion, there is no substitute for the mock patient encounter with a dedicated study partner: That's a must and makes more sense than buying any additional books.

REVIEW COURSES

How about review courses?

Here's a rundown on some of them:

1. *Kaplan 1-Day USMLE Step 2 CS Simulated Exam — Kaplan Cost: $999*

A close-to-the-real-thing simulation where each participant will take direct histories, perform focused physical exams, and write patient notes. This course, which is presently being offered at Mt. Sinai Medical Center in New York City and Stanford Hospital in Palo Alto, California, includes five standardized patient encounters conducted under exam conditions. At the end of the day, you will receive an analysis of your performance based on checklists completed by the standardized patients you have met during the encounter.

2. *Kaplan 5-Day Prep USMLE Step 2 CS — Kaplan Cost: $2699*

A comprehensive program providing hands-on review on skills assessed in the actual exam. This culminates in a 10-station practice examination. Presently being held in three locations: Chicago (Illinois), Palo Alto (California) and Rutherford (New Jersey).

3. *Kaplan Step 2 CS Practice Exam   Cost: $999*

   This course allows the examinee to experience what an actual Step 2 CS is like. Presently being offered at Kaplan Medical's Training Center in Rutherford, New Jersey, the program consists of 15-minute encounters with 10 standardized patients, each with an additional 10 minutes for writing the patient notes. Feedback, analysis and score is provided at the end of the exam.

4. *Kaplan History Taking Workshop   Cost: $299*

   This is a four-hour, skills-based workshop being offered in various cities in the United States. It reviews the fundamentals of history taking and emphasizes the importance of obtaining a relevant history in a short period of time and how to avoid mistakes in the actual Step 2 CS exam.

5. *Kaplan 6-day USMLE Step 2 CS   Cost: $3199*

   A hard-core review presently being offered at Kaplan Training Center in Rutherford, New Jersey. The course features hands-on interactive learning tutorials through various patient encounters culminating in a full-day Step 2 CS practice test with case review, and a final full-day practice exam.

6. *USMLEWorld Step 2 CS Course   Cost: $50 for 30 days/$60 for 45 days/$70 for 60 days*

   This is an online course providing information on topics including physical examination (with video clippings), history taking, communications skills, counseling, patient notes and many other relevant topics. It includes 28 sample cases and 43 practice cases. However, no actual patient encounter is offered with this course.

7. *FALCON Physician Reviews — USMLE Step 2 CS   Cost: $1200 to 1500*

   Presently being offered in Dallas, Texas, this course offers review of data gathering and physical exam with various clinical case scenarios.

8. *PassTheCSA.com Clinical Skills Assessment Exam Preparation Course   Cost: $249*

   The name may not be relevant anymore but the course is still available and is being offered in various cities across the country. International courses cost $399 and are usually administered in New Delhi, India and London, United Kingdom.

TUTORIAL CD OR DVD

Are there any tutorial DVDs or CDs available?

The following is a list of available visual tutorials available.

1. *Connecticut Tutorials (DVD) $89*
   http://www.conntutorials.com/index.html

There is no charge for viewing the Connecticut Tutorials on line but for a better resolution and audio, you will need to order a full copy of the DVD.

2. *Textbook of Physical Diagnosis: History and Examination (with CD-ROM)* by Mark H. Swartz *$72.95*

This CD-ROM comes together with the textbook, and it features a video demonstration of the complete physical examination of a man and the breast and pelvic examinations of a woman. If you do not have a fast Internet access where you can get free video demonstrations online, then this CD is probably your best choice.

3. *Bates' Guide to Physical Examination & History Taking (Book + CD-ROM)* by Lynn S. Bickley, Peter G. Szilagyi *$72.95*

This textbook provides a foundation for learning physical examination and history taking with emphasis on procedures, interpretations, and common abnormalities. Numerous color and halftone illustrations are included. Excellent for medical school but not the best for Step 2 CS; borrow if you can.

OBSERVERSHIP

What should I do to get some actual clinical experience in the United States?

Do a clerkship if you are still in medical school or an observership if you have already graduated. An elective clerkship in the United States will give you a front-row perspective on the American healthcare system and will help you become acclimated to the kinds of doctor-patient relationships that exists in this country. It may be a little costly, though. When I did my clerkship in cardiology at Yale a few years ago, I paid $1,200 for each month of rotation (that included malpractice insurance). I stayed in a dormitory and I had to pay for that too, plus the food and the cost of transportation. Today, the cost is much higher. An observership is less expensive and some institutions will provide free lodging and free lunch.

Where can I get a list of institutions that offer observerships?

Refer to the Appendices at the end of this book which lists several U.S. hospitals and institutions that offer observerships. I am unaware of any book or commercial online sites that currently offer this information. Some sites claim to have this information for sale but be careful about dealing with those sites. To avoid identify theft, deal only with reputable sites or those that are recommended by friends.

Do residency programs offer observerships?

It depends. You can send a snail mail (e-mail is too informal) addressed to the program director of your prospective specialty program. Tell him/her your reason(s) why you want to do an observership. Then follow up with a phone call (if you are in the U.S.) or an e-mail (if you are outside the U.S.). The advantage of this is that you will get a "feel" of the program and the people ahead of time, which will help you decide if this is the right place for you. And if they liked your personality and enthusiasm, you can ask them for recommendation letters, even if you decide not to pursue the residency there.

Are institutions with residency programs my only choice for observership?

No. You can contact any practicing physician who will be willing to let you do this. The best way is to ask a friend (preferably somebody who is already doing a residency) or a relative to connect you with a doctor that he/she knows. Referral is very important in the U.S., often more important than the contents of a resume or a curriculum vitae. It is very difficult — now — in the post 9/11 era — to arrange this without a connection, especially if you are from a foreign country.

Chapter 3

Communication

"Words are, of course, the most powerful drug used by mankind."
— Rudyard Kipling

- **What are the things to remember when counseling a patient?**
- **How do I establish rapport with the patient?**
- **What are standardized patients?**
- **How can I improve my English proficiency?**
- **How do I say words in layman's language?**
- **If I have a patient who continues to talk about trivial matters, how do I tell him to stop?**
- **How do I greet the patient?**
- **How about calling a patient by his/her first name?**
- **What are false assurances?**
- **How do I empathize with the patient?**
- **What do I do when a patient talks too fast?**
- **Seated or standing: What is the proper way for an IMG to interview a patient?**
- **What are transitional statements?**
- **How do I deal with challenging questions?**
- **Are open-ended questions important?**
- **Does my English need to be perfect?**
- **How about eye contact?**

- **How do I cope with belligerent patients?**
- **How do I pace myself when I am nervous and anxious to finish everything in the allotted time?**
- **How do I deal with patients who try to seduce me?**
- **Any online resources that deal with doctor-patient communication issues?**

COUNSELING A PATIENT

What are the things to remember when counseling a patient?

The information must be clear.

It is important to gauge the patient's level of understanding regarding health issues. Some patients may have limited formal education but are conversant in health issues, especially those that affect them. Nevertheless, the information that you will pass on to them must not contain any jargon or misleading medical terms and must be clear, concise, understandable, unbiased and offered with sincerity. Do not hesitate to ask a patient if he/she understood you. It is equally important to know if the patient is willing to commit to your suggestion or advice. Because, if he is not, then explain to him why that is important. If he is still unwilling to do it, do not insist.

The physician's skill in giving the information.

This can be tricky. Sometimes the patient will claim to understand you, but deep inside, you feel that he or she does not. There are several techniques to confirm a patient's understanding of what you have said. First, ask the patient directly if what you have said makes sense. Second, you can ask the patient to repeat the information. Third, ask the patient if he/she has any questions about the information or advice that you have provided. Fourth, give a hypothetical scenario and ask him what he would do in such a case. And fifth, if applicable, ask him to demonstrate to you how he understood the information.

Encouraging questions.

There are situations when the patient's real problem comes up when he starts asking questions. For example, a patient who initially came in for depression might ask,

"Doctor, don't you think my problem has something to do with my diet or habits?" That opens the door for other possibilities like alcoholism or substance abuse. It is crucial to give patients the chance to ask questions, not only because it is important they understand you, but also because they want to bring something up.

Answering questions.

Another important issue is how you answer questions. They have to be answered in a way that the patient won't be made to feel ignorant. Answering a question the right way can help generate trust and may make the patient more comfortable in divulging what the real problem is.

Summarizing and connecting the information together.

The ability to connect the dots and present the information to the patient as a complete picture is a skill you should develop. This is like putting all the pieces of the puzzle together, and letting the patient see the complete scene. In a concise manner, wrap the chief complaint, history of present illness, and physical examination together and tell the patient your clinical impression. This will portray you not only as an organized person, but as a skillful practitioner as well.

Explaining the course of action.

Be very clear in what you intend to do, what you want the patient to do, and what you and your patient expect to do in future encounters. For example, at the end of your interview, tell the patient, "Mr. Jones, I will be ordering some blood tests to check your cholesterol. Be sure that you fast for at least 10 hours before they draw your blood. During your next visit, I will be discussing with you what the result from the tests tell us and we will go from there."

A clear and appropriate use of language.

Most foreign medical students worry about this issue. You would do well to remember that what matters most is that patients understand you and you understand them. Regardless of your accent or your comfort level with English, encourage the patient to interrupt you if there is something he does not understand. Say something like this, "Mr. Jones, if you do not understand anything I've said because of my accent, please do not hesitate to stop me and ask for an explanation."

ESTABLISHING RAPPORT

How do I establish rapport with the patient?

Be attentive and do not rush.

Listen to what your patient is saying and do not interrupt unless he obviously veers from the main issue. Try to make the interview process go smoothly without long pauses. Short pauses are acceptable and may even be necessary at moments when you want to give the patient some time to gather his thoughts. Avoid asking questions the way journalists ask politicians during news conferences — the so-called "rapid fire" questions. The patient will know if you are rushing, and will consequently feel that you are not concerned enough about his welfare. Pace yourself in a manner that will help the patient feel you are giving him your attention, care and compassion.

Use appropriate body language

Good eye contact, appropriate facial expression, your position during the interview, your gestures, your body reaction as the patient talks. These are examples of body language that will help the patient feel comfortable. You can nod your head or use hand gestures if you want the patient to continue. Shrugging your shoulder, scratching your head, wrinkling your forehead, and smiling inappropriately are examples of body language that can make the patient feel uncomfortable. Your eyes should be at the same level with the patient so you may have to stand up if the patient is seated on the examining table. Too much body movement will cue the patient that you are nervous and not confident in what you are doing.

Be honest but sensitive.

Generally, Americans are candid. Many expect their physicians to tell them exactly what their condition is. Americans also value courtesy and expect other people to do likewise. Being direct and sensitive at the same time can be challenging, but it is definitely doable. It means you must say things tactfully. Use your judgment during the conversation and never give any false assurances or premature diagnosis. Do not hesitate to admit you do not know an answer if you are asked about something you are not certain about. Reassure the patient that you will provide him with an answer at the next appointment. Say something like, "Mr. Jones, that is a subject I am not familiar with, but I will provide you with the answer the next time you come to see me."

Show empathy.

Put yourself in the patient's shoes. Verbally and/or physically show that you care and understand your patient's concerns. You can say things like, "I can understand your concern" or "That must have been very difficult for you." Sometimes you may have to touch a patient's hand or gently pat his back.

Understand the implications of the patient's illness.

You can ask the patient how he feels about his illness. Sometimes, it may be necessary for you to inquire about his lifestyle, or the availability of a family member to assess the impact of the illness on his way of living, and/or to determine the adequacy of his social support system.

STANDARDIZED PATIENTS

What are standardized patients?

Also called SPs, these are people who are paid to act as patients and portray the physical signs of a disease. They know the signs of the disease they are asked to simulate, and are knowledgeable about the different physical exams you ought to perform during an exam. They have a checklist, which they fill out after you leave the room. That checklist can include your English proficiency, rapport, communication and history gathering skills, and the completeness of the physical examination. You will be evaluated based on the tasks you performed, the questions you asked, and your professionalism, as enumerated on the checklist. Some SPs have the physical signs or disease they are asked to mimic — but you won't know which ones are acting and which ones are authentic. Treat each patient as an authentic patient.

ENGLISH IMPROVEMENT

How can I improve my English proficiency?

Step 2 CS is meant to gauge a doctor's ability to communicate with a patient. And it carries a sizeable amount of English language component. Your English doesn't have to be perfect, but you must be able to speak in a manner that will be understood by a typical American patient. Although TOEFL assesses a foreigner's English proficiency just the same, Step 2 CS goes further by evaluating it in a clinical perspective. Being able to do well in this category will bolster your final score.

If you are not confident with your English language skill, attend classes offered by colleges in your area. Sylvan prometric offers classes to improve your English; visit the company's website at *prometric.com* for more information. If you are too busy to attend classes, buy English language tapes, listen to them and practice on your own. Talk to Americans as often as you can, so you can become familiar with their accents and their idiomatic expressions.

LAYMAN'S LANGUAGE

How do I say words in layman's language?

You will have to explain it in a way that a typical American can understand. The following are examples of medical jargons and their equivalent in layman's language:

Anemia = low blood count
Anorexia = loss of appetite
Abdomen = belly / tummy
Auscultate = listen to
Arthralgia = joint pains
Barium enema = taking a special liquid which will let us take a picture of the inside of your belly
CBC = blood test that will count and classify the cells
CXR = x-ray or picture of your chest
Constipation = difficulty in passing stools / difficulty pooping
Coitus = sexual intercourse
CVA = stroke
Endoscopy = a tube that will let us see your food passages and your stomach
ECG = machine that will test your heart
Enzymes = special proteins

Edema = swelling
Epistaxis = nosebleeds
Hemorrhage = bleeding
Hypertension = high blood pressure
HCG = pregnancy test
Inflammation = redness and pain
Insomnia = difficulty falling asleep
DVT = clotting problems in the blood vessels
Ecchymosis = bruising
Leukemia = cancer of the blood
Urinalysis = urine exam
Glucose = blood sugar
Vomit / vomitus = throw up
Syncope = pass out / faint
Nausea = sick to the stomach
Tinnitus = ringing in the ears
Odynophagia = pain while swallowing
Pallor = paleness
Tachycardia = rapid heartbeat
Polydipsia = excessive thirst
Urine = pee
Polyuria = pee a lot
Polydipsia = drink a lot
UTI = bladder infection
Veins / arteries = blood vessels
GIT = food passages
Respiratory tract = air passages
Lipid profile = test for body fats
Stool = poop
Sputum = spit
Cervical lymphadenopathy = bumps in the neck
Tumor = bumps or lumps
Mammography = x-ray of the breast
Spasm = muscle tightening
Orthopnea = sleeping with more than 2 pillows
Trauma = severe injury
Peripheral edema = swelling in the ankle, leg or foot
MI = heart attack
Regurgitation = back flushing
Melena = black stools
Tenesmus = urgency to poop
Vertigo = dizziness
Urticaria = itchy skin

Jaundice = yellowing
Pruritus = itchiness

Refer to the Appendices for a thorough list of medical words and their corresponding layman's words.

OTHER COMMUNICATION ISSUES

If I have a patient who continues to talk about trivial matters, how do I tell him to stop?

An SP can do this on purpose to test your diplomatic skills. This is a good way of gauging your ability to communicate in a way that won't be too harsh, yet still straightforward. The key to this is by saying it in an amicable and diplomatic tone, yet honest and straight to the point. Try this, "Mr. Jones, I understand that you have a very interesting life, and you would like to talk about it but for now, we need to focus on your immediate concern so let's go back to the headache you were telling me about."

How do I greet the patient?

The safest way to do this is to call a male patient — Mr. (and his last name) and a female patient Ms. (and her last name). In many countries, the proper and polite form of salutation is based on a person's age, social or marriage status. In the United States, calling a married person Ms. (instead of Mrs.) is fine, but it is different the other way around. Some female patients might get offended if they are unmarried and you call them Mrs. So it is safer to call every woman patient Ms.

In some other countries when you are talking to a person much older than you, you have to use "ma'am" for females and "sir" for males. You don't just say "yes" or "no" but you to say "yes, ma'am" or "yes, sir." In the U.S., you won't be branded impolite if you don't do this. You can answer a patient's question with a straight "yes" or "no" without the salutation. Minimize the use of "sir" or "ma'am."

How about calling patients by his/her first name?

Ask your patients what they prefer to be called. Say, "Do you prefer to be called, Mr. Jones or John?" Patients will often reply, "It doesn't matter to me." In many countries, you can call people by their first names only if they are about your age or younger. Calling an older person by his first name is tantamount to disrespect. In the U.S., you can call a 65-year old woman Rose or an 85-year old man Henry. If you don't feel comfortable doing this, then just refer to Rose as Ms. Adams or Henry as Mr. Smith. Note, however, that addressing patients can vary by region. In some parts of the U.S., addressing a patient by first name and/or by an incorrect salutation (Ms. or Mrs.), would be considered impolite.

What are false assurances?

These are statements you might inadvertently utter during the course of the discussion, and which will reduce your score. False assurances are statements like, "Don't worry, everything will be all right." "There is nothing to worry about." "Surely, it's not cancer." Statements such as these are inappropriate and should not be made.

How do I empathize with the patient?

Empathy is putting yourself into the other person's shoes. This is a skill every physician must possess in order to effectively establish rapport and build confidence. In the U.S., the way you empathize is very much the same way as in other countries — in words and in deeds — with few minor differences. Here, you can touch the patient's hands unlike in other countries. Here, I see some physicians hug their patients to console them in cases of tragedy. Gently tapping the shoulder or the back can also be a way of showing you care. If you come from a country where acts like these are considered inappropriate and you feel awkward doing them, you can still show you care and understand their situation by using the right words. For example, if the patient starts crying while telling her story, you can say, "I am sorry to hear that, Mrs. Jones. I do understand your situation. What do you do to cope with this?" Or you can say, "It must have been very difficult for you, considering your situation."

What do I do when a patient talks too fast?

Stop the patient, diplomatically. Something like this, "Excuse me for interrupting you, Mrs. Jones, but it will help me if you'll slow down a bit so I don't miss anything."

Seated or standing: What is the proper way for an IMG to interview a patient?

It depends. What feels comfortable to you? Just be practical. If you sit on a chair, adjust the seat to a level where you can see the patient's eyes. Or at least close to that level if you can't do it exactly on the same level. If you deem it more appropriate to stand up and do the interview, it is all up to you. Just make sure you both don't feel uncomfortable.

What are transitional statements?

These are statements you will use when you shift from one related set of questions to another. These statements make your interview less confusing to the patient and will reveal how organized you are. For example, after you have asked the patient about his present illness and you want to start asking him about his family and past medical history, you should start by saying, "Mr. Jones, since you've answered all my questions regarding these recent palpitations that you have been complaining about, now I will be asking you some questions about your past medical history and questions about illnesses in the family, alright?" Review the sample encounters in this book and note the various transitional statements used for each encounter.

How do I deal with challenging questions?

Challenging questions may range from the scientific to the mundane — just as in real life. Your response should be confident and honest. The physician must exude confidence to help earn the patient's trust and trust relates to compliance. Honesty should also play a key role. If a patient asks you something you know you've seen in Robbins during your sophomore year in medical school but have forgotten, be forthright in saying that you do not know or admit that you are not familiar with the subject. Offer to review and discuss it with him at a later time. Your response should not be condescending or humiliating to the patient.

It's not unusual for patients to search the Internet and have information about their particular condition prior to seeing a physician. Don't be caught off guard when patients come prepared with information and with questions. Try saying something like this, "I'm glad you did a lot of reading on the subject. It's been a while since I have encountered this and a lot has changed since then. But I will be willing to sit down with you and discuss these things when you come back for your next visit."

Are open-ended questions important?

Yes. Ask open-ended questions as often as you can. Your interview will provide you with more information if you use this technique. SPs are trained to spot them so give them what they want. Some questions may have to be asked using close-ended questions but these won't give you points. Patients tend to be more cooperative if they can talk a little more freely than just saying yes or no. Besides, some symptoms simply lurk in the dark and they only come out when patients start talking.

Does my English need to be perfect?

No. Although communication carries a huge bulk of the grade, language is just a part of it. Good communication eye contact, rapport, empathy, body language, plus a lot more. Your English doesn't need to be perfect, but patients do need to be able to understand you. You can have a heavy accent and still pass the Step 2 CS, provided patients understand what you say and you, on the other hand, understand what the patients say. It helps if you are fluent in English but don't be discouraged if you are not; your grammar doesn't have to be flawless, either.

How about eye contact?

In some countries, looking people in the eye is a sign of disrespect. In the U.S., if you don't look at the person you are talking to, it may be perceived as a sign of insincerity or people will think you are hiding something. It can also mean you are discourteous. Make eye-to-eye contact so patients will know that you are serious and sincere.

How do I cope with belligerent patients?

By maintaining your cool. That's when training comes into play. You must maintain your composure amidst the pressure. SPs are trained to gauge your convincing power and your decision-making skills by intentionally being uncooperative and verbally aggressive. Use a dialogue that will encourage the patient to calm down. Explain that you are there to help him. Do not get irritated; if you do, don't show it. He's there to test you. He can be belligerent throughout the entire process but be patient and continue on. Focus your exam on his presenting complaints. Rule out thyroid disorders, substance abuse or psychiatric problems. Some patients may calm down after you have said the right words and have struck the right chords. But expect for others to give you a full 15 minutes of nightmarish experience.

How do I pace myself when I am nervous and anxious to finish everything in the allotted time?

Psyche yourself up that this is just another day in your life as a physician. Your efforts will be fruitless if you rush things. The patient will notice if you are in a rush and may, in turn, refuse to cooperate with you, eventually compounding your problem. Do the history gathering and the physical examination in a normal, unhurried way. It is expected and understandable if you are anxious or nervous during your first or second encounter, but you are expected to relax as you continue through the exam. It is important that you simulate the time restrictions during your mock encounters with a study partner. By doing so, you will become familiar with the setup and will have at least an idea if your pacing is up to par or not.

How do I deal with patients who try to seduce me?

Be straightforward. Tell the patient that you are there to fulfill your job in a professional manner. But do so in a diplomatic tone. These are situations where your ethics will be tested. Don't ever fall into the trap. You went to the United States to take an exam — not for a fishing expedition.

ONLINE RESOURCES

Any online resources that deal with doctor-patient communication issues?

Here are some online sites you can refer to:

American Academy of Physician and Patient (AAPP)

http://www.physicianpatient.org

The AAPP is a professional society that promotes high standards for physician-patient communication. This site provides valuable information on how this can be achieved.

Communication Skills Program: Dalhousie Medical School

http://www.medicine.dal.ca/medcomm/strategies/index.htm

Covers important topics in developing effective communication skills including the management of angry patients, breaking bad news and appropriate communication techniques needed while performing the physical exam.

MedlinePlus

http://www.nlm.nih.gov/medlineplus/patientissues.html

A site providing a layman's perspective on issues pertaining to physician-patient communication.

NOAH-Patient Rights Resources and Physician Information

http://www.noah-health.org/english/patients.html

Tackles relevant issues regarding patients rights which might be useful especially for IMGs who are not familiar with the healthcare system in the United States.

NYU Macy Initiative on Health Communication, New York University

http://nyumacy.med.nyu.edu

Contains texts and videos that can enhance communication between doctors and their patients.

Patient Communications

http://www.patientcommunications.com

Contains links to various sites dealing with communication issues.

Program in Communication and Medicine, Northwestern University

http://www.pcm.nwu.edu/ipc/index.html

Offers abstracts to articles relating to physician-patient communication issues.

Chapter 4

Chief Complaint

"Orthodox medicine has not found an answer to your complaint.
However, lucky for you, I happen to be a quack."
— Richter cartoon caption

- **What is the chief complaint?**
- **How do I write the chief complaint on the patient note?**
- **How do I ask questions about the patient's chief complaint?**
- **What are the most common chief complaints that I will encounter in the clinic?**

What is the chief complaint?

The main symptom or chief complaint is the most important component of your assessment. It is the reason why the patient comes to you for help and your overall strategy will be based largely on this.

How do I write the chief complaint on the patient note?

You can write it as cc: followed by the clinical problem.

For example:

cc: shortness of breath
cc: chest pain
cc: diarrhea

Sometimes it can be written in the patient's own words:

cc: "feels useless"
cc: "feels tired all the time"

How do I ask about the patient's chief complaint?

Start by asking the patient what brought him in. This question is probably the most important question that you will ask the patient because it is where you elicit the chief complaint. Your history, physical examination, differential diagnosis and your lab work-up will all be based on the patient's presenting complaint so be keenly aware of his primary concern. Give him the freedom to describe or express what he is feeling. Interrupt him only if he starts veering from the main topic or if you need clarification.

Oftentimes, patients will give you a non-specific time period like "several hours ago" or "few months ago." These must be clarified. The term "several" or "few" can mean 3 hours to one person and 24 hours to another. For example, if the patient said, "I had chest pains several hours ago," you should ask exactly or approximately how long ago it was.

Inform the patient beforehand that you will be taking notes while he talks. If you don't explain this to patient, he might assume you are only listening half-heartedly. Say something like, "Mr. Jones, I will be writing some notes while you talk to be sure I don't miss any important detail in your story." This will assure the patient that you are paying close attention to his condition and demonstrating your commitment to details. This will help put him at ease and may help make him more comfortable in answering your questions.

What are the most common chief complaints that I will encounter in the clinic?

Here are the 35 most common complaints typically encountered in the clinics in the United States:

1. Headache	19. Visual Loss
2. Chest Pain	20. Hearing Loss
3. Abdominal Pain	21. Ear Pain
4. Knee Pain	22. Forgetfulness (Alzheimer's Disease)
5. Shortness of Breath	23. Difficulty of Urination
6. Fatigue	24. Substance Abuse
7. Frequent Falls	25. HIV
8. Diarrhea	26. Palpitations
9. Syncope/Seizure	27. Pallor
10. Menstrual Cramps	28. Spousal Abuse
11. Routine Physical Examination	29. Amenorrhea
12. Photosensitivity	30. Depression
13. Eye Pain	31. Joint Pain
14. Dysphagia	32. Schizophrenia
15. Polyuria	33. RLQ Pain
16. Back Pain	34. Pediatric Patient
17. Rash	35. Left Flank Pain
18. Sore Throat	

Chapter 5

History of Present Illness

"Nature has given to man one tongue, but two ears,
that we may hear from others twice as much as we speak."
— Epictetus

- **What is the History of Present Illness?**
- **Can I write while the patient is telling his story? Is this ethical in the United States?**
- **How should I write it in the patient notes?**

What is the History of Present Illness?

This is the patient's story — the patient's statements on how the chief complaint came about. It opens the door to information which you will gather and sort through. Be aware that the patient may not give you a chronological list of events that transpired prior to his consultation with you so it is your responsibility to guide him through this. Repeat his statement, if necessary, and ask him if what you said is accurate or you can ask him directly which event came first, which came second, and so on. When you interrupt, explain that you want to clarify something and be sure that you say this in a way that won't offend him or make him think that you are not paying attention. What he tells you in this section will determine what maneuvers you will perform in the physical exam and what further tests you will be ordering.

Can I write while the patient is telling his story? Is this ethical in the United States?

You have to let the patient know that you will be jotting down notes while he is telling his story. Mention that you do not want to miss any important information that will help you in assessing his condition. This is an accepted practice in the United States and patients will not feel that you are incompetent.

The Step 2 CS bulletin states that you will be provided with a blank sheet you can use to write down patient data during the interview. Do not spend too much time writing. Abbreviate everything you can and write only the relevant ones. You could lose points in your communication skills even if your data gathering was superb but the patient thought you were more interested in perfecting your notes than attending to his needs.

How should I write it in the patient notes?

The notes may be written in a narrative or outline. Either form is acceptable as long as the notes are legible.

Below are examples of both a narrative and an outline format.

Narrative format:

HPI: 18 y/o female soccer player c/o knee pain that started 4 days ago after a gym practice. Described as continuous, knife-like, exacerbated by walking or standing and relieved by non-usage. No medications taken aside from Tylenol every 4 hrs since yesterday which afforded temporary relief. Severity is 6/10 in the pain scale.

Outline format:

HPI:
- *18 y/o female soccer player*
- *c/o knee pain that started 4 days ago after a gym practice*
- *continuous, knife-like*
- *exacerbated by walking or standing; relieved by non-usage*
- *no meds taken aside from Tylenol q 4 hrs since yesterday, afforded temporary relief*
- *severity: 6/10 in the pain scale*

Chapter 6

Past Medical History

"The past is the best prophet of the future."
— Lord Byron

- **What is the Past Medical History?**
- **How do I ask questions about the patient's past medical history?**
- **How do I ask patients about medication intake?**
- **How do I ask questions about allergies?**
- **How do I ask questions about their diet?**
- **Can you give examples on how this is written in the patient notes?**

What is the Past Medical History?

This is the record of the patient's previous hospitalizations, childhood or adult illnesses, glucose level, cholesterol level, surgeries, trauma, date of most recent physical exam, date of most recent procedure or lab tests (e.g., mammogram, PSA). Many institutions include the medication, allergy or dietary history as part of the PMH while others want them written separately on another line.

Allow the patient to provide you this information voluntarily. However, if there is something he missed and you feel that information is relevant to the case, do not hesitate to ask specific questions.

How do I ask questions about the patient's past medical history?

Start by asking the patient if he has been hospitalized before or if he has had any illnesses that took him longer than usual to recover from.

For example, "Mr. Jones, have you been hospitalized before?" or "Did you have any illnesses in the past that took you longer than usual to recover from?" Sometimes, patients will respond "no" initially but upon further questioning would remember they had measles in childhood or an allergic reaction to seafood.

If the patient can't give you an answer with an open-ended question, try a direct one by asking him if he ever had any accidents, injuries, high blood sugar, etc. — questions that can be answered "yes" or "no." Again, be selective in asking only about those diseases or injuries that you think would be relevant to your initial impression.

How do I ask patients about medication intake?

You can ask them, "Are you taking any medication right now?" Many American patients are well aware of the doctor-prescribed medication they are taking. Compared to other countries where medications like steroid-containing skin ointments, certain antibiotics, oral contraceptive pills and others can be bought over the counter without a doctor's prescription. In the United States, in contrast, most of these drugs are not available without a prescription yet cold medications, drugs for fever, pain, diarrhea or heartburn are widely available in most U.S. pharmacies and are sold over the counter. Take note that some patients may presume that these are not the medications you are asking for, so make sure that you use the word "any" to refer to all prescription and over-the-counter medications.

How do I ask questions about allergies?

Ask them if they are allergic to anything. If they are unsure, ask them if they ever had any rashes, sneezing, or difficulty breathing after eating certain foods, after taking certain medications, or after being exposed to animals.

How do I ask questions about their diet?

Generally, a typical American diet consists of high-fat, low-fiber foods, which account for the staggering number of obese and hypertensive patients — not to mention those that have colon cancer. You can ask this question if you think your initial impression demands it.

Can you give examples on how this is written in the patient notes?

Example 1:

PMH: no h/o of allergies, hospitalizations or accidents

Example 2:

PMH: hospitalization for heart attack 5 yrs. ago, no other similar episode since then; no allergies, no accidents, no h/o surgery

Chapter 7

Other Relevant History

"Good friends, good books, and a sleepy conscience; this is the ideal life."
— Mark Twain

- **What is a Family History?**
- **How do I gather data for family history?**
- **Can you give examples on how this is written in the patient notes?**
- **What is a Social History?**
- **How do you ask personal or sexual questions in ways that won't offend the patient?**
- **How do I ask for a social history in a professional and American way?**
- **Can you give examples on how this is written in the patient notes?**
- **Any suggested online resources for doing a basic sexual history interview?**
- **What is a Menstrual and Obstetrical History?**
- **How do I obtain a menstrual or obstetrical history?**
- **Can you give examples on how this is written in the patient notes?**
- **When is the developmental history necessary?**
- **Can you briefly summarize the pediatric developmental milestones?**

FAMILY HISTORY

What is a Family History?

This is a record of the patient's information regarding the medical conditions of the other family members which include the father, mother, brothers, sisters, spouse and children. Genetic diseases will also be included in this section.

An SP may offer irrelevant information like a distant cousin's arthritis problems or the grandfather's visual problems in an attempt to waste your time. Tactfully tell the patient that you do not find this information relevant and guide him toward a more meaningful discussion.

How do I gather data for family history?

This is a straightforward interview. You inquire about the past or present occurrence of a particular disease in the family on both the father's side and the mother's side. Also, ask for the same thing about siblings and/or offspring. Ask something like this, "Does anyone in your family have diabetes? How about kidney disease?" Focus your questions on relevant disease entities that will help you evaluate his condition.

Can you give examples on how this is written in the patient notes?

Example 1:

FH: mother has HTN, father has diabetes

Example 2:

FH: – father died of heart disease
– brother has knee pain with fever at present

SOCIAL HISTORY

What is a Social History?

This is a record of the patient's social status, children, occupation, living arrangements, use of cigarettes, alcohol, recreational drugs and sexual orientation.

How do you ask personal or sexual questions in ways that won't offend the patient?

Ask the questions in a professional way. Do not use jargon. Use simple words they can understand. Make an introduction before you start asking them questions about their lifestyle. For example, "Mr. Jones, I will be asking you some questions which I feel are important in making a complete assessment of your medical condition. These can be about your sexual history or personal lifestyle. I just want to assure you that your answers will be kept confidential. Is that okay with you?" If patient consents, begin with your questions. Be careful when doing this. If the patient is offended by the way the question is asked, apologize and restate the question in a different way. Refer to the sample encounters in this book that deal with these issues.

How do I ask for a social history in a professional and American way?

Be diplomatic, non-judgmental and honest. For example, if you want to find out if the patient is taking drugs or not, do not ask him, "Mr. Jones, do you take drugs?" Instead you can say, "Mr. Jones, I will be asking you some personal questions regarding your lifestyle which will help me better evaluate your medical condition. You can be assured that your answers will be kept confidential. Is that ok with you? Have you taken any prohibited drugs in the past? Are you taking any of these at present?"

Another aspect of social history that may be difficult to obtain is sexual orientation or preference. In this case, offer the same introductory statement as you did with the question on drug abuse, assuring the patient of confidentiality, and that the patient's answer will help you in your overall health assessment. Never ask a patient directly if he or she is homosexual, heterosexual or bisexual. Ask something like this, "Have you had any sexual encounters in the past with a person of the same sex? How about at present? Do you prefer having sexual relations with a man, a woman or both?" This way, the patient won't feel intimidated and may be less hesitant in divulging his lifestyle or sexual preferences.

The other components of the social history will be easy to elicit. Marital status, social support system, occupation, alcohol and smoking history can all be asked in a direct manner.

Can you give examples on how this is written on the patient notes?

Example 1:

SocH: *cig (–), etoh (–), illicit drugs (–)*
sexually active with husband only, no h/o STD
works as a truck driver

Example 2:

SocH: *– doesn't exercise, drinks alcohol 1–2 cups/week*
– sedentary lifestyle, cig (–), drugs of abuse (–)

Any suggested online resource for doing a basic sexual history interview?

These websites may be of help:

University of Virginia: A Basic Sexual History

http://www.med-ed.virginia.edu/courses/pom1/videos/basic-sexual-hist.cfm

This features a short video that introduces a way of performing or gathering information about a patient's sexual history. The three-minute video may require Quicktime.

University of Virginia: A Focused Sexual History

http://www.med-ed.virginia.edu/courses/pom1/videos/focused-sexual-hist.cfm

This video, also from the University of Virginia, provides an example of how to interview patients on matters related to sexual issues.

MENSTRUAL AND OBSTETRICAL HISTORY

What is a Menstrual and Obstetrical History?

This is a record of the female patient's information which include the last menstrual period (LMP), GP score, pregnancy status, age of menarche, age at menopause, last Pap smear, contraception, menstrual characteristics, childbirth, and sexual problems.

Eliciting this information may sometimes provide difficult, especially if the patient cannot remember exactly when she had her LMP or when her most recent Pap smear was done but be patient in gathering this data. Be familiar with the GP score because if you are pressed for time, the GP score alone will provide a lot of information regarding the patient's status.

How do I obtain a menstrual or obstetrical history?

You have to ask the female patient about her last menstrual period (LMP). You also have to make sure that a female patient is not pregnant before you order an x-ray. This part of the history can be very important. The OB score is also helpful because it gives information about the patient with only a few characters, which won't crowd the very limited space on your patient note sheet. If the presenting symptoms of a female patient point to a menstrual or gynecological disorder, you may need to elicit more information than only the LMP and the OB score.

Can you give examples on how this is written in the patient notes?

Example 1:

OB/GYN H: menarche at 13 y/o, menopause at 43 y/o
Pap smear 2 years ago with normal result
G2P2

DEVELOPMENTAL HISTORY

When is the developmental history necessary?

Developmental milestones are important pieces of information that should be included in the patient notes when you are dealing with a pediatric case. Cases such as these seldom appear in the Step 2 CS but being prepared for such a scenario can mean the difference between passing or failing.

Can you briefly summarize the pediatric developmental milestones?

2 months	–	coos, head lags, follows objects visually
4 months	–	rolls, reaches with 2 hands, brings objects to midline
5 months	–	sits with trunk support, transfers objects from one hand
6 months	–	sits, reaches with one hand, babbles vowels, stranger anxiety
7 months	–	crawls
8 months	–	creeps, says "Dada"
9 months	–	throws objects, pincer function, says "Mama," holds bottle
10 months	–	separation anxiety
12 months	–	stands, walks with help, utters 2 other words, "jargoning"
15 months	–	crawls up stairs, utters 6 words, puts up 2 blocks, hugs, uses spoons & cups, scribbles lines
18 months	–	two-word combo, makes strokes, partly feeds self
2 years old	–	says "no," makes 7 blocks, uses pronouns, does parallel play
3 years old	–	three-word combo, feeds self, undresses, draws circle/cross/square
4 years old	–	joint play, colors, toilet trained, hops, skips, catches ball, dresses self, draws person
5 years old	–	follows rules, helps in tasks, draws triangle, prints name, ties shoes, counts

Chapter 8

Review of Systems

"How unfair! Only one health, and so many diseases."
—Victor Schlichter

- **What is the Review of Systems (ROS)?**
- **How do I do the ROS systematically?**
- **Do I have to be thorough in doing the Review of Systems (ROS)?**
- **How do I ask the ROS questions?**
- **Can you give examples on how the ROS is written in the patient notes?**

What is the Review of Systems (ROS)?

This is a record of the patient's symptoms based on the different body systems including general review, HEENT, respiratory, cardiovascular, gastrointestinal, genitourinary, musculoskeletal, integumentary, neurological, endocrine, and psychological.

How do I do the ROS systematically?

I find it easy and organizationally efficient if I do a head-to-toe review of systems in much the same way I do a physical examination. Others will find it easier to do it based on the various systems method. Choose the method that suits your style and use it consistently so you won't get disorganized during the exam.

Do I have to be thorough in doing the Review of Systems (ROS)?

Being thorough is different from being complete. Having a complete list of a patient's symptoms from head to toe is not only impractical in the Step 2 CS but also next to impossible. With just a few minutes to do the history, physical examination and closing statements, it is imperative that the ROS gathering be focused. A thorough review of the patient's relevant symptoms is what's needed. Be selective with the questions you ask the patient. Be systematic. You can do a head-to-toe approach, choosing only those symptoms you deem appropriate with your initial impression or you can do an organ system approach. It's up to you. Do whatever you are comfortable with and always keep in mind that Step 2 CS is meant to test your proficiency in selecting what is relevant and what is not.

How do I ask the ROS questions?

Below are sample scripts you can use when doing the ROS. These are suggested scripts — you have to use whatever you are familiar with and you find comfortable.

Constitutional Symptoms:

1. How is your health in general?
2. How is your energy level?
3. Do you have difficulty sleeping?
4. Do you feel tired when you wake up in the morning?
5. How is your appetite?
6. How is your weight? Have you noticed any recent changes in your weight?
7. Do you have a fever? Does you whole body shake?
8. Do you have night sweats?

Skin

1. Do you have any problems with your skin?
2. Any itching?
3. Do you bruise easily?
4. Do you bleed easily?
5. Any moles that have recently changed color or size?
6. Do you have any ulcer, sores or wounds that don't heal?
7. Do you have problems with your hair or nails?

Head

1. Did you hurt your head?
2. Did you pass out? For how long?
3. Do you feel lightheaded or dizzy?
4. Do you have a headache?
5. Do you feel any spinning sensation?

Eyes

1. Do you wear glasses?
2. When was your last eye exam?
3. Do you have any trouble with your eyes?
4. Do you feel any pain in your eyes?
5. Have you noticed any changes in your vision?
6. Any blurring or double vision?

7. Did you notice any redness? Any itchiness? Any discharge? Any excessive tearing?
8. Do you see any flashes, spots or floaters?
9. Do you see halos around lights?
10. Do you find it difficult to adjust your vision from dark to light?

Ears

1. Do you have any trouble with your ears?
2. Do you have trouble hearing things?
3. Any pain? Any discharge?
4. Do the insides of your ear itch?
5. Do you hear ringing in your ears?

Nose

1. Any problem with your nose?
2. Any discharge coming out of your nose?
3. Any nosebleeds?
4. Do you have problems with your sinuses?

Mouth and Throat

1. Any problems with your mouth or throat?
2. Any toothaches? Cavities?
3. Do you have dentures?
4. Any sores or ulcer on your tongue or in your mouth?
5. Do you have any trouble chewing or swallowing?
6. Any sore throat?
7. Have you noticed any changes in your voice?

Neck

1. Any complaints about your neck?
2. Does your neck feel stiff?
3. Does it hurt anywhere in your neck?
4. Do you feel any bumps on your neck? Are they painful?

Respiratory

1. Do you have any problem breathing?
2. Any cough? Does it produce any gunk? What color? How often does this happen?
3. Can you walk without resting?
4. How many flights of stairs can you climb without stopping?
5. Do you have trouble breathing when lying on your back?
6. How many pillows do you use when you sleep?
7. Do you hear a wheezing sound when you breathe?
8. Do you feel any pain when you breathe?

Cardiovascular

1. Do you have any trouble with your heart?
2. Do you feel any pain in your chest? Does the pain spread?
3. What does the pain feel like?
4. Did the pain occur at rest or after exertion?
5. Any problem with your heartbeat?

Gastrointestinal

1. Do you feel nauseous? Did you vomit? What did it look like? Was there any blood?
2. Any heartburn? Do you feel like the acid in your stomach backflushes to your throat?
3. Do you have pain in your belly? How do you describe the pain?
4. Do you have diarrhea? What did your stool look like? Was it soft or hard? What was the color? Was there any blood?
5. Do you have trouble with constipation?
6. Did you have black or tarry stool?
7. Have you noticed any change in the frequency of your bowel movement?
8. Have you noticed any change in the caliber or size of your stool?
9. Do you have hemorrhoids? Is there something coming out of your rectum?
10. Have you noticed any changes in your skin color? (jaundice)

Genitourinary

1. Do you have any trouble peeing?
2. Does it burn when you pee?
3. Are you peeing more frequently than usual?
4. How often do you pee at night?
5. Do you notice any color changes in your urine?
6. Do you have any problem starting your urine?
7. Do you have any problem stopping your urine?
8. Does your urine leak when you cough or sneeze?
9. Do you feel like you need to use the bathroom in a hurry?
10. Have you noticed any change in the size or force of the stream?
11. Do you feel like there is still some urine in your bladder after you pee?

Reproductive (Female)

1. Do you have any discharge from your vagina? Any itching?
2. Have you noticed any warts, sores or ulcers around your vagina?
3. When did you start getting your periods? Do you get them regularly? How many days between periods? How long do they last? How many pads/tampons do you use? Are they mildly, moderately or fully soaked?
4. When was your last menstrual period?
5. Do you have painful periods?
6. Do you notice any change in the amount of your periods?

7. Do you have any bleeding between periods?
8. Do you notice a change in yourself physically or emotionally several days before you get your period?
9. Have your periods stopped?
10. Any hot flashes?
11. Are you in a sexual relationship now?
12. Are you in a sexual relationship with a person of the opposite sex, or the same sex or both?
13. Do you find your sexual relationship fulfilling?
14. Do you have any problem reaching an orgasm?
15. Have you noticed any loss of interest in sex?
16. Do you feel pain during sexual intercourse?

Reproductive (Male)

1. Have you noticed any warts, sores or ulcers on your genitals?
2. Do you have any unusual discharge?
3. Do you have any pain or swelling in your testes?
4. Do you have a hernia?
5. Are you in a sexual relationship right now?
6. Are you in a sexual relationship with a person of the opposite sex, or the same sex or both?
7. Do you find your sexual relationship fulfilling?
8. Do you have trouble maintaining an erection?
9. Do you have any trouble controlling ejaculation?

Breast

1. Any problems with your breasts?
2. Do you check them regularly for lumps?
3. Does it hurt anywhere in your breasts?
4. Any discharge from the nipple?
5. Have you noticed any skin changes on your breasts?

Musculoskeletal

1. Do you have pain in your legs (or arms)?
2. Does the pain occur when you are doing something or when you are at rest?
3. Do you have swollen or painful joints?
4. Do you have any joints that feel stiff? At what time of the day do they usually feel stiff? How long do the stiffness last?
5. Do you have back pain?

Endocrine

1. Do you have trouble adjusting to a temperature in a room? Do you prefer it warm or cold?
2. Do you feel like you are thirsty all the time?

3. Do you feel like you want to pee all the time?
4. Have you noticed any changes in your hair recently?
5. Have you noticed any changes in the size of your shoes or hat?

CNS

1. Do you have any problem with your smell?
2. Do you have any problem with your taste?
3. Do you have any problem with your vision?
4. Do you feel any weakness in your arms or legs?
5. Do you feel any weakness in moving the muscles of your face?
6. Do you feel any numbness anywhere in your body?
7. Do you feel any unusual sensation anywhere in your body? How would you describe it?
8. Are you bumping into things — frequently?
9. Are you dropping things more often than usual?
10. Do you have any trouble maintaining your balance? Are you falling more frequently than usual?
11. Do you have any problem walking?
12. Do you have any unusual shaking or jerking movements?
13. Do you have convulsions or fits?
14. Do you have trouble remembering things?
15. Do you have any problem focusing?
16. Do you have any trouble talking, reading or listening?
17. Do you feel relaxed or anxious most of the time?
18. Do you feel sad?
19. Have you ever thought of hurting yourself or others?

Before proceeding to Physical Examination

1. Anything else we haven't covered?
2. Do you have any problems you'd like to focus on?

Can you give examples on how the ROS is written in the patient notes?

Example 1:

ROS: Respiratory, cardiovascular, GI, and endocrine are unremarkable

Example 2:

ROS: Repiratory: (+) dyspnea, (+) wheezing
Cardiovascular: no palpitations, no murmur
Neuro: no loss of consciousness

Chapter 9

Physical Examination

"Physical examination must be carried out with a watchful eye, a sensitive touch, discerning ears, and an alert sense of smell."
— Maxwell Wintrobe

- **What am I expected to do in the Physical Examination?**
- **Do I have to repeat the vital signs when they've been done?**
- **Any online resources where I can review issues pertaining to vital signs?**
- **What is covered in the general appearance?**
- **How do I perform an HEENT exam?**
- **Are we required to do fundoscopy or otoscopy when doing the physical examination?**
- **Any online resources where I can review issues pertaining to the proper performance of the HEENT exam?**
- **What is covered in the neck exam?**
- **Any online resources where I can review issues pertaining to the proper performance of the neck exam?**
- **How do I perform a respiratory exam?**
- **Any online resources where I can review issues pertaining to the proper performance of a respiratory exam?**
- **How do I perform a cardiovascular exam?**
- **Am I allowed to do inguinal node or femoral pulse exam?**
- **If I need to do a thorough chest exam on a female patient, do I ask her to remove her bra?**

- **Any online resources where I can review issues pertaining to the proper performance of a respiratory exam?**
- **How do I perform an abdominal exam?**
- **Any online resources where I can review issues pertaining to the proper performance of an abdominal exam?**
- **How do I perform a genitourinary exam?**
- **Am I allowed to do inguinal node or femoral pulse exam?**
- **How do I perform a musculoskeletal exam?**
- **Any online resources where I can review issues pertaining to the proper performance of a musculoskeletal exam?**
- **How do I perform a neurological exam?**
- **In neuro cases, are we expected to do all the neuro exams?**
- **Do I need to do the physical examination in psychiatric cases?**
- **Any online resources where I can review issues pertaining to the proper performance of a neurological exam?**
- **Can you give an example on how I should write the physical examination findings in the patient note?**
- **What does an ordinary doctor's office look like in the United States?**
- **How do I introduce myself? Should I shake hands?**
- **When should I wash my hands — before or after examining the patient?**
- **How important is washing hands before doing the physical examination?**
- **When do we drape patients?**
- **If I accidentally drop an instrument on the floor, what will I do with it?**
- **After washing my hands, what if the room has no paper towels?**
- **What will I do if a patient is not wearing a gown and I want to do a physical examination?**
- **During the physical examination, how can I be relevant and thorough at the same time?**
- **How do I make the patient comfortable when doing the physical examination?**
- **What if the patient becomes belligerent or uncooperative during the physical examination?**
- **What are the restrictions in doing the physical exam?**
- **I feel uncomfortable examining a white, female patient in a gown. What should I do?**

- **I want to get refreshed in doing a proper physical exam. Is the Step 2 CS video enough as a review?**
- **What do you do if a patient comes in for a routine check-up without any complaints?**
- **How do we handle pediatric cases? Are we going to get actual pediatric patients?**
- **How about geriatric patients?**
- **15 minutes is such a short time to do everything. Can I look at my watch every once in a while during this 15-minute period?**
- **How do you handle belligerent patients?**
- **Any other resources that offer tutorial in doing the physical exam?**

PRACTICE CHECKLIST

What am I expected to do in the Physical Examination?

You are expected to perform all maneuvers learned from medical school. Below is a checklist of the most common exams you can review and perform with a study partner. You are expected to be proficient in performing these exams.

Physical Examination Checklist:
(Put a check after performing each test with a study partner.)

Vital Signs:

☐ 1. Blood Pressure
☐ 2. Heart Rate
☐ 3. Respiratory Rate
☐ 4. Orthostatic Changes

Head:

☐ 1. Hair loss

Eyes:

☐ 1. Visual Acuity
☐ 2. Extraoccular muscle (EOM) functions
☐ 3. PERRLA
☐ 4. Ophthalmoscopic exam

Nose:

☐ 1. Palpate and percuss sinuses

Ears:

- [ ] 1. Auditory Acuity
- [ ] 2. Rinne's Test
- [ ] 3. Weber's Test
- [ ] 4. Otoscopic exam
- [ ] 5. BPPV evaluation

Mouth:

- [ ] 1. Inspect mouth, tongue and throat
- [ ] 2. Tongue deviation
- [ ] 3. Hypoglossal nerve function
- [ ] 4. Gag reflex
- [ ] 5. Uvular deviation

Neck:

- [ ] 1. Lymph node palpation (post auricular, submandibular, cervical, supraclavicular)
- [ ] 2. Thyroid
- [ ] 3. Tracheal position and mobility
- [ ] 4. Neck ROM (range of motion)
- [ ] 5. Jugular venous distention
- [ ] 6. Carotid bruits

Anterior Chest:

- [ ] 1. IFDA (inspection, fremitus, dullness, auscultation — in that sequence!)
- [ ] 2. PMI palpation and auscultation
- [ ] 3. Heart sounds (4 positions, valsalva or inspiration — if indicated)

Posterior Chest:

- [ ] 1. IFDA
- [ ] 2. Diaphragmatic excursion
- [ ] 3. CVA tenderness
- [ ] 4. Breath sounds

Axilla:

- [ ] 1. Lymph nodes

Abdomen:

- [ ] 1. IAPP (inspection, auscultation, percussion, palpation — in that order!)
- [ ] 2. Bowel sounds (one quadrant)

- ☐ 3. Bruit (2 sides)
- ☐ 4. Percussion (4 quadrants)
- ☐ 5. Hepatomegaly evaluation
- ☐ 6. Splenomegaly evaluation
- ☐ 7. Light and deep palpation (4 quadrants)
- ☐ 8. Rebound tenderness
- ☐ 9. Hepatic tenderness
- ☐ 10. Hepatojugular reflux
- ☐ 11. Shifting dullness
- ☐ 12. Psoas sign
- ☐ 13. Obturator sign
- ☐ 14. Rovsing's sign
- ☐ 15. Cough or jarring test for acute appendicitis
- ☐ 16. Murphy's sign
- ☐ 17. Cullen's Sign
- ☐ 18. Grey-Turner's sign

Pulses:

- ☐ 1. Carotid, brachial, radial
- ☐ 2. Femoral, popliteal, posterior tibial, dorsalis pedis

Nervous:

- ☐ 1. MMSE
- ☐ 2. 12 cranial nerves (motor and sensory)
- ☐ 3. Reflexes (biceps, triceps, knee, Achilles tendon)
- ☐ 4. Motor functions (upper and lower extremities)
- ☐ 5. Heel to knee
- ☐ 6. Finger to nose
- ☐ 7. Rapid alternating movements
- ☐ 8. Heel to toe
- ☐ 9. Cogwheel rigidity
- ☐ 10. Brudzinski's sign
- ☐ 11. Kernig's sign
- ☐ 12. Get up and go
- ☐ 13. Babinski
- ☐ 14. Hoffman's sign

Upper Extremities:

- ☐ 1. Motor, sensory and reflexes
- ☐ 2. Tinel's sign
- ☐ 3. Phalen's sign
- ☐ 4. Allen's test

Lower Extremities:

- ☐ 1. Motor, sensory and reflexes
- ☐ 2. Anterior Drawer test
- ☐ 3. Homan's sign
- ☐ 4. Filament test

Hips:

- ☐ 1. ROM

Spine:

- ☐ 1. ROM
- ☐ 2. Gait
- ☐ 3. Romberg's
- ☐ 4. Test for sciatic irritation
- ☐ 5. Test for disk herniation
- ☐ 6. Straight leg raising test
- ☐ 7. Test for Scoliosis

Note: Genitourinary, pelvic, rectal, female breast examinations, inguinal hernia assessment, and corneal reflex are not to be performed in the USMLE Step 2 CS. If the presentation and clinical history demand such performance, order them as part of work-ups.

VITAL SIGNS

Do I have to repeat the vital signs when they've been done?

Vital signs, as mentioned in the USMLE information bulletin, are usually posted on the door together with the chief complaint. It is not necessary to repeat them unless you question the posted result. For example, if the respiratory rate were written as 16 cycles per minute but the patient is obviously having tachypnea, you may have to repeat the vital signs.

Any online resources where I can review issues pertaining to vital signs?

University of Virginia Health System

http://www.med-ed.virginia.edu/courses/pom1/videos/vitals.cfm

A comprehensive video series demonstrating the process of obtaining a patient's pulse, respiratory and blood pressure. You will need Quicktime and a high-speed Internet connection.

GENERAL APPEARANCE

What is covered in the general appearance?

The patients age, race, alertness, orientation (in person, time, place), well-developed or otherwise, well-nourished or otherwise, in apparent distress or not.

HEENT

How do I perform an HEENT exam?

Assess the head, hair, scalp and note any abnormalities. Evaluate the eyes and pupils by various maneuvers and by ophthalmoscopy. Check the visual acuity with Snellen's chart, if applicable. NEVER DO A CORNEAL REFLEX EXAM! Assess the ears by otoscopy and by doing Rinne's and Weber's tests. Inspect the nose for discharge or bleeding, mucosal color, nasal septum abnormality. Look at the throat and oral cavity, lips, palate, tongue, tonsils, teeth, gums, and gag reflex.

Are we required to do fundoscopy or otoscopy when doing the physical examination?

In the official Step 2 CS video (now available online), you will notice that these instruments will be at your disposal. It is all up to you — just like in real life. If you think this will aid you in making a correct diagnosis, then why not? Just make sure it won't take a big bite out of your very limited time. If you are dealing with an ophthalmology or otolaryngology case, you definitely will have to use them. In other cases, use them arbitrarily. If it has been a while since you've done any of these procedures, try practicing these procedures with a study partner. The SPs will most likely note if you know how to use them or have actually used them in their particular case. The Step 2 CS bulletin states that SPs will only grade the encounter. In other words, just use them, if necessary, even if the last time you have touched one was when Margaret Thatcher was still the Prime Minister of the U.K.

Any online resources where I can review issues pertaining to the proper performance of the HEENT exam?

Eye Simulation Application

http://cim.ucdavis.edu/EyeRelease/Interface/TopFrame.htm

This site provides an eye motion and pupil response simulator, animations to demonstrate neurological testing, and quizzes to test comprehension. It also provides a set of patient cases with various neurological pathologies and a multiple-choice quiz that assesses comprehension from the topics covered. Requires Shockwave plugin (Version 8 or greater) and Quicktime (Version 4 or greater).

The Ophthalmoscopic Exam

http://www.med-ed.virginia.edu/courses/pom1/videos/ophthalmoscopic.cfm

This basic-level video from the University of Virginia features a demonstration and explanations on how ophthalmoscopic exam is done. You will need high-speed Internet connection.

Basic Clinical Skills: Head, Eyes, Ear, Nose and Throat Exam

http://imc.gsm.com/scripts/mainframeset.asp?url=http://www.imc.gsm.com/integrated/bcs/index.html

This site, available for a fee, claims it is designed to decrease variability in the teaching of physical diagnosis, and to provide an ongoing resource for the learning of these skills. The program includes over 150 illustrations, over 200 photographs, video, sound, and more than 300 pages of content with links to glossary terms.

Online Otoscopy Tutorial

http://www.uwcm.ac.uk:9080/otoscopy/index.htm

High-resolution video describing the anatomy of the ear and demonstrating the proper technique of conducting an otoscopy.

University of Virginia: HEENT Exam

http://www.med-ed.virginia.edu/courses/pom1/videos/HEENT.cfm

An excellent video showing scalp inspection, visual field testing, ophthalmoscopy, Rinne test, Weber tests, and oral exam.

Virtual Eye Clinic

http://www.homeusers.prestel.co.uk/academy/reception.htm

A virtual simulation where a user can practice data collection and diagnosing eye problems.

Basic Eye Exam PowerPoint Slides

http://medinfo.ufl.edu/year2/clinmed/ppt/basic_eye_exam.html

A Powerpoint presentation on basic ophthalmologic exam.

NECK

What is covered in the neck exam?

You assess the trachea, larynx, thyroid, carotid artery, jugular venous distention (JVD), and range of motion (ROM).

Any online resources where I can review issues pertaining to the proper performance of the neck exam?

Thyroid Exam

http://www.lumen.luc.edu/lumen/MedEd/MEDICINE/PULMONAR/PD/pstep24a.htm

This is a useful site from Loyola University consisting of a discussion on the appropriate steps of a thyroid exam. Includes a self-evaluation questionnaire but no video or simulation is included.

RESPIRATORY

How do I perform a respiratory exam?

Check for breath sounds like rales, rhonchi, wheezing, etc. Assess the chest contour, resonance, diaphragmatic excursion and paradoxical movement. Proper performance of a chest exam requires the strict sequential execution of inspection, fremitus, dullness and auscultation which is often referred to as IFDA.

Any online resources where I can review issues pertaining to the proper performance of a respiratory exam?

The R.A.L.E Repository

http://www.rale.ca/

Various recordings of normal and abnormal lung sounds available in Real Audio or WAV formats. Most are free but a more comprehensive commercial software is available for purchase.

Screening Physical Exam — Pulmonary Exam

http://www.meddean.luc.edu/lumen/MedEd/medicine/pulmonar/pd/contents.htm

This site from Loyola University offers a systematic approach to conducting a pulmonary exam which includes tracheal palpation, chest inspection, voice transmission, lung percussion and auscultation. The texts are culleted for easy reading with still images and videos that clearly demonstrate the steps covered in the texts. Another feature of this site is the inclusion of normal and abnormal breath sounds which would be of value to those who have been out of the clinic for some time.

The Chest Exam

http://www.med-ed.virginia.edu/courses/pom1/videos/chest.cfm

This video is a section from the University of Virginia website with a demonstration on the proper way of doing a lung and heart exam with an excellent discussion at each step of the exam. The video quality is excellent but no heart or lung sounds are available and high-speed Internet connection is required.

Respiratory Examination

http://www.medinfo.ufl.edu/year1/bcs/clist/resp.html

This is a portion of the physical examination study guide from the University of Florida website. No video and few images but provides an organized and easy to follow outline of doing the pulmonary exam which includes inspection, palpation, percussion and auscultation.

The "Auscultation Assistant"— University of California, Los Angeles
http://www.wilkes.med.ucla.edu/intro.html
Covers topics including heart sounds, heart murmurs, and breath sounds for medical students and other health care professionals to help improve diagnostic skills.

CARDIOVASCULAR

How do I perform a cardiovascular exam?

By assessing rate, rhythm, murmurs, gallops, rubs and clicks. Also check for the point of maximum impulse (PMI).

Am I allowed to do inguinal node or femoral pulse exam?

These are not considered genital exams so you can perform them. But let the patient know beforehand what you intend to do and do it in a way that will not make them uncomfortable. Genital or rectal exams, on the other hand, cannot be performed on SPs but can be included or ordered in the work-ups. NEVER DO INGUINAL HERNIA EXAM. Again, if needed, order it as part of the work-ups.

If I need to do a thorough chest exam on a female patient, do I ask her to remove her bra?

Ask the patient if she will remove her bra and be very clear in letting her know what you wish to accomplish. Tell her that it is important that you get an unobstructed access to the area to make your findings more accurate. Some patients would prefer to have the hooks at the back unfastened without removing the bra. That also will work just fine. If the patient declines, do not insist. Honor her privacy. If she refuses to remove the bra, proceed with the examination. If you need to auscultate the chest, the flat or bell of your stethoscope must directly come in contact with the patient's skin. NEVER EXAMINE THROUGH THE GOWN.

Any online resources where I can review issues pertaining to to the proper performance of a respiratory exam?

Heart Sounds Tutorial
http://www.blaufuss.org/tutorial
A wonderful resource with animation of each valvular lesion and its corresponding heart sound.

FamilyPractice.com HeartLab Cardiac Auscultation Simulator

http://www.familypractice.com/heartlab/heartlab.htm

An excellent site allowing the user to listen to various heart sounds by clicking a particular area of the heart.

The Practice of Medicine: The Cardiac Exam

http://www.med-ed.virginia.edu/courses/pom1/videos/cardiac.cfm

A comprehensive high-resolution rendition of the proper execution of a heart examination including inspection, palpation, auscultation and assessment of pulses. Requires high-speed Internet connection.

Screening Physical Exam — Heart

http://www.meddean.luc.edu/lumen/MedEd/medicine/pulmonar/pd/contents.htm

Texts, still images and audio files of various heart sounds courtesy of Loyola University.

The Auscultation Assistant

http://www.wilkes.med.ucla.edu/inex.htm

Extensive collection of audio files containing various heart sounds from UCLA.

Howard Hughes Medical Institute Virtual Cardiology Lab

http://www.hhmi.org/biointeractive/cardiovascular/vlab.html

A computer simulation of a cardiology exam with tutorial.

Physical Exam Study Guides: Cardiovascular Examination

http://www.medinfo.ufl.edu/year1/bcs/clist/cardio.html

A text-only site providing methods for assessing arterial pulses, JVP, precordial movements and auscultation.

McGill University Virtual Stethoscope

http://sprojects.mmi.mcgill.ca/mvs/mvsteth.htm

Provides a tutorial for auscultation and other selected topics in cardiology and pulmonary physiology or pathophysiology.

Normal & Abnormal Heart Sounds & EKGs — Frontiers of Science

http://bioscience.org/atlases/heart/

Features EKG and various heart sounds encountered in normal and abnormal conditions.

Synapse Publishing

http://www.medlib.com/spi/coolstuff2.htm

A great online review of the various heart sounds.

ABDOMINAL

How do I perform an abdominal exam?

By performing a strict sequential execution of inspection, auscultation, percussion and palpation (IAPP). Also check for bowel sounds, bruit, hepatomegaly, splenomegaly, rebound tenderness, hepatic tenderness, hepatojugular reflux, shifting dullness, obturator sign, Rovsing's sign, Murphy's sign, Cullen's sign and Turner's sign. NEVER REPEAT ANY PAINFUL MANEUVER.

Any online resources where I can review issues pertaining to the proper performance of an abdominal exam?

Screening Physical Exam — Abdominal Exam

http://www.meddean.luc.edu/lumen/MedEd/medicine/pulmonar/pd/contents.htm

Another section from the Loyola University website providing an outstanding discussion and demonstration of how the abdominal examination is done which includes inspection, palpation (superficial and deep) including liver and kidney palpation and liver percussion. Although no videos are available, the quality of the images is good and the accompanying texts provide descriptions and information which are useful for the Step 2 CS.

The Abdominal Exam

http://www.med-ed.virginia.edu/courses/pom1/videos/abdomen.cfm

Another installment from the University of Virginia video series on doing the physical examination. This section shows a physician discussing and demonstrating the basic abdominal exam with great emphasis on the liver, spleen and kidney. High-speed Internet connection required.

GENITOURINARY

How do I perform a genitourinary exam?

This cannot be performed during the actual exam. It would have to be ordered as a part of the work-ups.

Am I allowed to do inguinal node or femoral pulse exam?

Yes. These are not considered genital exams so they can be performed. Inform the patient that you will be examining the inguinal area for pulse or bumps. Alerting the patient about what you plan to do next may help to create an atmosphere of trust and make the performance of the exam less intimidating. NEVER PERFORM AN INGUINAL HERNIA ASSESSMENT. This is not allowed in the exam.

MUSCULOSKELETAL

How do I perform a musculoskeletal exam?

By checking the muscles, bones and joints of the four extremities. Also check for ROM, swelling, atrophy, hypertrophy, spasm, motor, sensory and reflexes. Performance of special tests including Tinel's, Phalen's, Allen's, Homan's and anterior drawer test may be necessary in some cases.

Any online resources where I can review issues pertaining to the proper performance of a musculoskeletal exam?

The Practice of Medicine: The Upper Extremities

http://www.med-ed.virginia.edu/courses/pom1/videos/upextremities.cfm

A good, quality video demonstrating the proper way of conducting an examination of the upper extremities.

The Practice of Medicine: The Shoulder Exam

http://www.med-ed.virginia.edu/courses/pom1/videos/shoulder.cfm

A brief video clip showing the correct procedure in assessing the shoulder.

The Practice of Medicine: The Lower Extremities Exam

http://www.med-ed.virginia.edu/courses/pom1/videos/lowextrem.cfm

Another outstanding video from the University of Virginia showing the proper protocol in performing the passive range of motion of the hip, ankle and knee.

Musculoskeletal Exam

http://www.lumen.luc.edu/lumen/MedEd/MEDICINE/PULMONAR/PD/musc.htm

Provides a refreshing review of how to perform a musculoskeletal exam courtesy of Loyola University.

NEUROLOGIC EXAM

How do I perform a neurological exam?

Check for mental status, orientation, memory, abstract reasoning, speech, cranial nerves, motor, sensory and reflexes.

In neuro cases, are we expected to do all the neuro exams?

Use only those that you think would be appropriate. You must remember that some neuro cases have concomitant cardiovascular components. Spending too much time on the neuro without looking at the other possible scenarios would be detrimental and the question of relevance takes center stage. Ask yourself if the test you are going to perform will add credence to your initial impression or not. Use your analytical skills. Decide what you think is right for each case.

Do I need to do physical examination in psychiatric cases?

The mainstay of psychiatric cases is the MMSE (mini mental status exam). You must be a pro at doing this. Performing actual physical maneuvers will strongly hinge on your initial impression. For example, in cases of depression, aside from the MMSE, you also need to rule out thyroid disorders, Parkinson's or even anemia. So, you have to check the thyroid gland, do a cogwheel rigidity test or gait test, or look at the insides of the eyelids for pallor. Also, be on the lookout for physical or substance abuse in these cases. It all depends on how you analyze the case. That is what the Step 2 CS is all about — to determine if you know what is relevant and what is not.

Any online resources where I can review issues pertaining to the proper performance of a neurological exam?

NeuroLogic — An Anatomical Approach to the Neurological Exam

http://medstat.med.utah.edu/neurologicexam

An excellent site containing texts, still images and good, quality videos prepared by an antomist and a neurologist. The site focuses on correlating neuroanatomy with the normal and abnormal neurological exams. Emphasis is placed on assessing the patient's mental status, cranial nerves, motor and sensory deficits, and coordination and gait. It also has a section on how to do neuro-developmental exam in pediatric patients.

Neurological Examination

http://icarus.med.utoronto.ca/NeuroExam

Combining texts and high-quality video, this site provides a comprehensive demonstration on how to perform the neuro examination with emphasis on cranial nerves, motor exam, sensory exam, stance and gait.

NeuroExam.com

http://www.neuroexam.com

This is an interactive online guide to the neurologic examination, with video demonstrations intended for medical students, residents, and other students in the health care professions. It complements "The NeuroExam Video" which is offered for sale but a video demo is available for free and both can be viewed by using a 28.8 modem or high-speed Internet connection.

Central Nervous System Exam

http://www.lumen.luc.edu/lumen/MedEd/MEDICINE/PULMONAR/PD/cns1.htm

This site features still images accompanied by descriptions and diagrams that will facilitate a quick understanding and retention of the fundamentals in conducting a neuro exam.

The Neurological Exam

http://www.med-ed.virginia.edu/courses/pom1/videos/neuro.cfm

Another excellent video clip demonstrating the proper performance of a neuro exam including the assessment of the cranial nerves, motor, sensory and reflexes. You will need a high-speed Internet connection.

Can you give an example on how I should write the physical examination findings in the patient note?

Below is an example of how physical examination findings can be written.

Physical Examination

General: A&O X3, cooperative, not in acute distress

VS: BP: 120/80 HR: 80 RR:16 T: 38.6 C

Head: normocephalic, normal hair distribution, no scalp tenderness, no rashes, no tumors

Eyes: PERLA, EOM intact, fundi WNL, sclerae clear, normal convergenge, no pallor, no proptosis, normal visual activity with reading glasses

Ears: normal otoscopic findings BL, can appreciate whisper at 3 ft., membrane intact BL, no discharge, Weber midline, Rinne negative

Nose: no nasal discharge or bleeding, normal mucosal color, nasal septum midline

Mouth: tongue midline c N size, color & texture; no ulcers or tumors; no buccal or pharyngeal erythema; no bleeding gums, tonsils not enlarged, no whitish plaques

Neck: no lymphadenopathy (cervical, postauricular, supraclavicular, occipital), no JVD, trachea midline, no carotid bruit, no thyroid enlargement, tenderness or nodules

Chest/Lungs: symmetrical BL, N breath sounds BL, normal vocal & tactile fremitus, no dullness, clear breath sounds BL, no rales, no egophony, no wheezes

Breast (if applicable): symmetrical c no masses or erythema, no abnormal bleeding or discharge, normal skin color & texture

Heart: N rate, regular rhythm, PMI not displaced; no murmurs, gallops, rubs or clicks; no S3/S4 noted

Abdomen: slightly rounded c no scars, NBS X4 quadrants, no organomegaly, no tenderness, no guarding, tympanitic to percussion, no tenderness on light & deep palpation X4 quadrants, no palpable mass, (–) H/S megaly, (–) Murphy's, (–) Rovsings, (–) Psoas sign, (–) obturator sign

G-U: kidneys not enlarged BL, no CVA tenderness, no hernia, testicles descended with no tenderness, no abnormal bleeding or discharge

Ext: N muscle tone & strength, ROM not reduced, sensory intact, DTR normal, no tenderness, pulses palpable (femoral, popliteal, dorsalis pedis), no pedal edema, no clubbing, no cyanosis, (–) Homan's sign

Skin: normal color & turgor, no rashes, no tumors, no scars, no edema

Neuro: CN III-XII intact, (–) finger to nose test, 5/5 motor strength X4 extremities, ++ DTR X 4 extremities, sensory intact X 4 extremities, (–) Babinski

Mental: alert, conscious, oriented X3, normal behavior, speech fluid & goal-oriented, intact recent & remote memory, can do serial 7s, can spell "world" backward, mood is sad, affect consistent with mood, no illusion, no delusions, judgment not impaired, no suicidal or homicidal ideation

OTHER PHYSICAL EXAMINATION ISSUES

What does an ordinary doctor's office look like in the United States?

It can vary a bit from one place to another but it is standard to see an examination bed, a BP cuff, ophthalmoscope, otoscope, a sink, a paper towel dispenser, a small desk or table and a chair. You must be familiar on how to use the diagnostic instruments attached to the wall and how to adjust the bed so you won't look awkward when you need to use them.

There are three parts of the examining table that you must be familiar with. The knob for adjusting the head part of the bed, the sliding extension for the legs, and the sliding step that will make it easier for patient to get off or get onto the table.

Usually a set of disposable earpieces is available when you need to do otoscopy. Pull one earpiece from the bottom and twist it onto the otoscope. If it falls off, do not pick it up — use a new one. The otoscope can also be used like a penlight if you want to examine the throat, the nasal passage, or the pupil reaction to light and accommodation. Be sure to remove the earpiece when you do this. The other items you will need (tongue depressor, cotton, etc.) should be available either near the sink or on a table.

Some sample pictures of a standard doctor's office in the United States can be seen at the official USMLE website at *http://www.usmle.org*.

How do I introduce myself? Should I shake hands?

You can shake hands depending on the situation but introduce yourself to all patients. Shaking hands is the American way of greeting and it helps in "breaking the ice" and establishing rapport. It should show sincerity and not just simple formality. But if the patient is lying down, doubled up or wincing in pain, a simple introduction without the handshake would suffice. Use your judgment.

When should I wash my hands — before or after examining the patient?

I think this is the most important part of the physical examination. You are expected to wash your hands before touching any patient for examination. Sometimes you will be so preoccupied with the interview and exam process that at the end, you can't remember if you washed your hands or not. If this happens, wash your hands at the end of the exam. I personally believe that washing before and after each examination is mandatory. More importantly, you will prevent the spread of germs.

How important is washing hands before doing the physical examination?

Very important! You have to do this each time before you examine a patient. If you fail to do this, one crucial point will be deducted from your score. Sometimes, a point can either make or break you so make sure you do not miss this important part of the exam.

When do we drape patients?

Step 2 CS assesses how you honor the patient's privacy and comfort. When you ask the patient to lie down to be examined, place a drape on body parts that will be exposed. This will help keep them comfortable and will help assure them that you are a physician who values their privacy. Some patients may feel cold in a hospital gown, especially when they are seated on the examining table and their legs are dangling and uncovered. Ask them if they would feel more comfortable if you placed a drape on their legs.

If I accidentally drop an instrument on the floor, what will I do with it?

If it is disposable, throw it in the trash. If not, make sure that it is cleaned or disinfected before using it again. If you find no cleanser or disinfectant in the room, set it aside and put a note that instrument is dirty and needs to be cleaned. DO NOT USE IT UNLESS IT HAS BEEN CLEANED.

After washing my hands, what if the room has no paper towels?

Look for a clean drape and use it to wipe your hands. Do not open the door and tell the proctor that you are out of paper towels. NEVER LEAVE THE ROOM! Because once you step out of the room and the door closes, you will not be allowed to return. Just look for anything clean inside the room and use it. If nothing else is available, and you are running out of time, just use the inside of your lab coat but do this only as a last resort.

What will I do if a patient is not wearing a gown and I want to do a physical examination?

Ask the patient to change to a hospital gown. Gowns can come as disposables (paper gowns) or washables (cloth gowns). They are usually given to patients before you enter their rooms. If a patient hasn't changed into to a hospital gown, you may have to tell him that he needs to change to make the examination easier for him and for you. Typically, you would step out of the room while the patient changes but the Step 2 CS doesn't allow that. Once you step out of the room, you can no longer go back into the room. Explain to the patient that you will turn your back while he changes and ask him to let you know when he's changed so you can proceed with the examination. American examination rooms often have a privacy curtain, which will allow patients to change without you leaving the room.

During the physical examination, how can I be relevant and thorough at the same time?

Step 2 CS gauges your clinical skills. The skill of determining which ones are relevant and which ones are not are developed during clerkship and internship. This is the skill that Step 2 CS wishes to measure. Relevant means that you only do maneuvers that you think is appropriate to your initial impression. For example, if you suspect anemia, check the eye for pallor or the abdomen for possible bleeding or growth. Doing a fundoscopy or otoscopy, checking for cranial nerve deficit may not be relevant in this case. Thorough means that you have to perform all the necessary maneuvers that will shed light on your case. For example, if you're entertaining a possible case of depression, you do a psychiatric work-up and check the thyroid or check for signs of anemia.

How do I make the patient comfortable when doing the physical examination?

Always lend a hand when necessary. If you ask the patient to lie down, support his back or his head with your hand as he lies down. If you ask him to sit up, assist him in getting up. Do likewise if he needs to get out of the bed in case you want to test his gait or balance.

In addition, let him know what you intend to do before you actually do it. For example, before you auscultate his chest, tell him, "I will be listening to your chest." Make sure your stethoscope or your hands are not too cold. If your stethoscope is cold, rub it against your gown or with the palms of your hands to warm it up. If your hands are cold, warm it up in the faucet before touching the patient's skin. Before you tap the belly, inform him what you intend to do. In doing so, you will help make the patient feel at ease and cooperative.

What if the patient becomes belligerent or uncooperative during the physical examination?

This is seen in the clinics everyday. Such actions test your skills as a communicator and as a decision maker. Be on the lookout for psychiatric disorders, substance abuse, spousal abuse, metabolic disorders or other medical conditions that can make a patient behave abnormally. Always maintain your composure and talk in a diplomatic manner so as not to antagonize him.

Another thing to consider is to make sure that your technique is not hurting the patient. You might be bending his swollen osteoarthritic knees too much or you might be strongly tapping on an inflamed area. Informing him ahead of time what you intend to do minimizes bad encounters like these.

What are the restrictions in doing the physical exam?

No genitourinary, pelvic, rectal or breast exam for female patients. No inguinal hernia assessment and no corneal reflex exam. They all can be ordered as part of the work-up plan if you think they are relevant to your case. Checking for inguinal pulse is not a genital exam so that can be done. Lifting the breast to feel the heartbeat is not a breast exam so that can be done too but you should explain to the patient what you will be doing and why.

I feel uncomfortable examining a white, female patient in a gown. What should I do?

Don't be. Treat her as you would any other patient. Some Asian cultures harbor a Caucasian superiority complex. This perception can spill over in the clinics where they expect a Caucasian patient to be demanding or intimidating, particularly if the examining physician is a male and the Caucasian patient is a female. To some examinees, this may be your first time to see a Caucasian female patient in a hospital gown, and you may feel uncomfortable and hesitant in doing all the physical examination maneuvers. This should change if you aspire to do your residency in the states. Treat each patient with dignity and respect, regardless of their gender, and do not be intimidated.

I want to get refreshed in doing a proper physical exam. Is the Step 2 CS video enough as a review?

The tape is an overview of how the test is administered but it is far from perfect in covering a thorough physical exam. If you have access to a medical school library in the U.S., you can borrow videotapes that comprehensively deal with this subject matter. If you don't, you can scan the web and look for videotapes created for nurse practitioners and physician assistants (instructional) because these tapes can be a very useful resource. If you have high-speed Internet connection, you can use the sites mentioned in this book.

What do you do if a patient comes in for a routine check-up without any complaints?

Do a thorough interview and physical exam. This can be very tricky because you only have 15 minutes to do everything. Just like an actual patient, he may not have any medical complaints initially but as you go along the interview, you may unearth some hidden symptoms and you must be quick to start focusing on them. Don't forget to ask for weakness, weight changes, fever, etc. Listen to the chest and tap his abdomen. Ask for thyroid symptoms. Make quick relevant exams from head to toe. Try to inject a few psychiatric questions to rule out malingering. Such a situation like this is tough since you are going up against time. But it is certainly doable.

How do we handle pediatric cases? Are we going to get actual pediatric patients?

According to the official USMLE website, pediatric cases will be conducted over the phone. Instead of a pediatric patient in the room, expect to see a telephone. The person calling in will be a parent or a relative of a child seeking consultation for their child who is at home or too sick to come to the hospital. Obviously, in this case you cannot do a physical exam but you can put it as part of your further work-ups. The history should be expanded and more comprehensive because the entire15 minutes will be devoted to the interview.

How about geriatric patients?

As with pediatric patients, these "exams" will be conducted over the phone, as mentioned in the USMLE information bulletin.

15 minutes is such a short time to do everything. Can I look at my watch every once in a while during this 15-minute period?

If you look at your watch too often during the course of the interview, patients may think you are more interested on your watch than on their condition. You should remember that they are the ones grading your performance. Some Step 2 CS online forum participants suggest placing the face of your watch towards you, so you can make quick glances at it without the patient noticing it. Make sure you follow the Step 2 CS guidelines regarding watches.

How do you handle belligerent patients?

By maintaining your cool. That's when training and preparation come into play. You must keep your composure despite the pressure. Sometimes, even actual patients try to gauge your convincing power and your decision-making skills by intentionally being uncooperative and verbally aggressive. Use well-thought-out statements that will help persuade him to calm down. Explain that you are there to help him. Do not get irritated and if you do, don't show it. Patients can be belligerent throughout the entire process but be patient and continue on. Focus your exam on his presenting complaints. Rule out thyroid disorders, substance abuse or psychiatric problems. Some patients may calm down after you have said the right words and have struck the right chords. Expect for others to behave differently.

ONLINE PHYSICAL EXAMINATION RESOURCES

Any other resources that offer tutorial in doing the physical exam?

University of Virginia: Physical Exam/Interviewing Videos

http://www.med-ed.virginia.edu/courses/pom1/videos/index.cfm

These excellent videos cover examples on how to do the following: upper extremities exam, shoulder exam, vital signs, chest exam, abdominal exam, HEENT exam, lower extremities exam, cardiac exam, ophthalmoscopic exam, neurologic exam, and a basic sexual history. You will need high-speed Internet connection and Quicktime; the video clips vary from three minutes to seventeen minutes.

Harvard Medical School: NetNote!

http://www.asp.md/netnote/nn4/asp/welcome.asp

NetNote helps you write clinical notes and was intended for use by medical students. From the home page, click on "Medical Student" and a form will open which you can fill out and print on you own computer. NetNote does not transfer any information you enter into it over the Internet (all information remains on your local machine).

University of California-San Diego: A Practical Guide to Clinical Medicine

http://medicine.ucsd.edu/clinicalmed/introduction.htm

Provides a comprehensive discussion and great pictures covering the following topics: Write Ups, History of Present Illness, Male Genital/Rectal Exam, The Oral Presentation, The Rest of the History, The Upper Extremities, Exam of the Abdomen, Outpatient Clinics, Vital Signs, The Lower Extremities, Inpatient Medicine, The Eye Exam, The Mental Status Exam, Clinical Decision Making, Head and Neck Exam, The Neurological Exam, The Lung Exam, Exam of the Heart, Commonly Used Abbreviations, Putting It All Together.

Ohio State University Interactive Learning Center

http://medicine.osu.edu/exam

This is an interactive web-based learning center designed to teach medical students the fundamental principles of physical examination. Physician content specialists and web developers are using state-of-the-art, web-portable technologies to bring the sights and sounds of the physical examination alive. The primary content areas covered are the head and neck, pulmonary, cardiovascular, abdominal, musculoskeletal, neurological, male and female genitalia. This collection contains more than 45 digital video clips and more than 45 colorful, interactive multimedia elements.

UCSD Catalog of Clinical Images

http://medicine.ucsd.edu/clinicalimg/Index.html

A wonderful online atlas of clinical images that can be found on physical examination. The images are divided into categories which include the following: Head-Neck, Eyes, Thorax, Upper Extremities, Abdomen, Genital/Rectal, Lower Extremities and Skin. This site will also be useful for those taking the USMLE Step 2 CK and USMLE Step 3.

The Connecticut Tutorials

http://www.conntutorials.com/video.html

These are physical examination videos created by the University of Connecticut, which can be viewed without charge from their website using Windows Media Player. High-speed Internet connection required. The site offers a commercial version of these videos in the form of a 3-hr. DVD for sale.

Screening Physical Exam

http://www.meddean.luc.edu/lumen/MedEd/medicine/pulmonar/pd/contents.htm

A comprehensive discussion on the proper steps in performing a physical examination. This site from Loyola University is well-organized with some still images which appear good but probably not as good as when you can see them on video from other sites. One advantage this site has is that you do not need a fast Internet connection to use it.

Chapter 10

Differential Diagnosis

"The diagnosis that is never thought of is seldom made."
— Anonymous

- **How do I make a differential diagnosis?**
- **What if I only have four differentials? Will I lose points if I only write down four?**
- **Do I need to come up with the right diagnosis?**
- **Please give examples on how the differential diagnosis is written on the patient notes.**

How do I make a differential diagnosis?

You are allowed to make five differential diagnoses based on the patient's presentation and on the physical examination. You have to be certain that the differentials you list can be correlated with the patient's signs and symptoms or you will lose points.

What if I only have four differentials? Will I lose points if I only write down four?

I do not believe so but make sure that those four you listed are very good ones.

Do I need to come up with the right diagnosis?

Step 2 CS is basically about the process and not the result. You can come up with an incorrect impression on a particular encounter and still get a good score because you are being graded on the process or what actions you took to come up with your impression. You will be scored high if you asked the questions you are expected to ask and if you performed the appropriate physical examination. These are the major components of the exam and your efforts should be focused on these.

Please give examples on how the differential diagnosis is written on the patient notes.

Enumerated below are some of the common disorders, the differential diagnosis and their appropriate work-ups:

Differential Diagnosis and Work-ups

Osteoarthritis	
1. RA	1. Rheumatoid factor
2. Septic Arthritis	2. Joint fluid analysis & culture/CBC
3. Gout	3. Serum Uric Acid
4. SLE	4. ANA, anti-Smith, anti-dsDNA
5. Lyme Dse	5. Lyme ELISA
(6. Dislocation/Fracture)	*(6. For dislocation or fracture order Joint X-ray or MRI)*
Migraine Headache	
1. Hypertension	1. Repeat BP
2. Meningitis	2. CSF analysis/CSF C&S
3. Glaucoma	3. Tonometry
4. Sinusitis	4. X-ray of sinuses
5. Temporal Arteritis	5. ESR
(6. Cluster Headache 7. Tension Headache 8. Brain tumor)	*(6. Brain CT scan)*
UTI	
1. Nephrolithiasis	1. Urinalysis/C&S if indicated
2. Pyelonephritis	2. CBC with diff/Renal CT scan
3. STD	3. C&S of discharge
4. PID (if female)	4. Pap smear (if female)
5. BPH (if male)	5. Rectal Exam (if male)

(+) CXR Lesion 1. Pulm TB 2. Lung CA 3. Hamartoma 4. Fungal (Coccidioides, Histoplasma) 5. Pneumonia	1. PPD 2. Chest CT scan/Repeat CXR 3. Sputum GS, AFB & Cult 4. Fungal Ab 5. CBC with diff
Memory Loss 1. Alzheimer's 2. Major Depression 3. Head Trauma 4. Substance/Alcohol Abuse (Korsakoffs Syn) 5. AIDS dementia	1. Lytes/B12 2. Drug screen 3. Alcohol level 4. HIV ELISA 5. Cranial CT or MRI
Hip Injury 1. Osteoporosis. 2. Pathological Fracture due to Tumor 3. Hip Joint Dislocation 4. Osteoarthritis 5. Polymyalgia Rheumatica	1. DEXA scan 2. Serum Ca^{++} 3. Hip X-ray 4. ESR 5. CBC
Fever with Cough 1. Pneumonia 2. COPD 3. TB 4. CHF 5. Lung CA	1. CXR/Sputum GS, C& S 2. PFT/H&H/ABG 3. PPD/Sputum AFB 4. EKG/Echocardiogram 5. Chest CT
GERD 1. PUD 2. Acute MI 3. Pericarditis 4. Pulmonary Embolism 5. Acute Pancreatitis	1. EKG/CK-MB/Troponin 2. Amylase/Lipase 3. D-dimer, V/Q scan 4. Esophageal ph monitoring/ Manometry 5. Endoscopy

Constipation 1. Low-fiber diet 2. Hypothyroidism 3. Colon CA 4. Hirschsprung's Disease 5. Electrolyte imbalance *(hypokalemia, hypercalcemia)*	1. TSH/FT4/T3 2. FOBT 3. Lytes/Calcium 4. Rectal Exam 5. Sigmoidoscopy/Rectal biopsy
Diabetic Neuropathy 1. Vit. B12 Deficiency 2. Beriberi or Alcoholic Neuropathy 3. Vascular Insufficiency 4. Drug-induced neuropathy-INH 5. Uremia *(6. Polyarteritis nodosa)*	1. FBS 2. Serum B12 3. Doppler ultrasound 4. BUN/Crea 5. Lytes *(6. HBsAg, p-ANCA)*
Child with Fever 1. Otitis Media 2. Meningitis 3. Bronchiolitis 4. Pneumonia 5. UTI	1. Physical Exam/ CBC/ Otoscopy 2. Blood Culture/ CSF analysis, C&S 3. RSV Ag 4. CXR/Sputum GS, C&S 5. Urinalysis with C&S
Cough (HIV + with Hemoptysis) 1. Pneumocystis Pneumonia 2. TB 3. Lung CA 4. Wegener's Granulomatosis 5. Pulm Embolism	1. CXR/ Sputum Giemsa or Methenamine Silver stain 2. PPD/Sputum AFB stain & Cult 3. Chest CT 4. c-ANCA 5. D-dimer, V/Q scan
Female Victim of Sexual Assault 1. Physical/Sexual Abuse 2. Domestic Violence 3. Generalized Anxiety Disorder 4. Substance Abuse 5. Borderline Personality Disorder	1. Genital exam 2. Pregnancy test/RPR/Pap smear 3. Wood's light for seminal fluid 4. Saline sample from mouth, anus, cervix 5. Pubic hair sample (obtained via combing)

Vomiting	
1. Gastroenteritis	1. Stool C&S
2. Intestinal Obstruction	2. Abdominal X-ray
3. Food Poisoning	3. ALT/Hepatitis screen
4. Hepatitis A or B	4. Amylase
5. Acute Pancreatitis	5. Lipase
(6. Pregnancy)	*(6. Serum B-HCG)*
Difficulty of Breathing	
1. Asthma	1. Pulse oxymetry
2. Pneumonia	2. Sputum GS with C&S
3. COPD	3. CXR
4. Pneumothorax	4. D-dimer, V/Q scan
5. Pulmonary Embolism	5. ABG
(6. Acute MI)	*(6. EKG/CK-MB/Troponin)*
(7. CHF)	*(7. Cardiac Doppler)*
Knee Pain	
1. Fracture/Dislocation	1. X-ray of the knee
2. Ligament Injury-Cruciate or Collateral	2. RF/ANA
	3. ESR
3. Osteoarthritis	4. Synovial fluid analysis and C&S
4. Rheumatoid Arthritis	
5. Gout	5. Serum uric acid
(6. Septic Arthritis)	*(6. CBC/Joint fluid analysis w/ C&S)*
(7. SLE)	*(7. ANA/ anti-Smith/anti-dsDNA)*
Fatigue	
1. Anemia	1. CBC
2. Hypothyroidism	2. TSH
3. Depression	3. FBS
4. DM	4. Lytes
5. Electrolyte imbalance	5. Iron/Ferritin/TIBC
Palpitations	
1. Hyperthyroidism	1. TSH
2. Panic Disorder	2. ECG
3. MVP	3. Echocardiography
4. Arrhythmia	4. Holter monitoring
5. Substance Abuse (Cocaine, caffeine)	5. Urine Drug Screen

Syncope 1. Vasovagal Hypotension 2. Arrhythmia 3. Hypoglycemia 4. Intracranial lesion 5. TIA	1. RBS 2. Recheck BP 3. Carotid duplex scan 4. Cranial CT 5. ECG
Rectal Bleeding 1. Hemorrhoids 2. Colon CA 3. Crohn's Disease 4. Ulcerative Colitis 5. Infectious Diarrhea	1. Rectal exam 2. CBC/Lytes 3. Stool analysis and C&S 4. FOBT 5. Sigmoidoscopy/biopsy
Check-up for Blood Pressure 1. Essential HTN 2. Pheochromocytoma 3. Diabetic Nephropathy 4. Renal Artery Stenosis 5. Conn's Syndrome *(6. Cushing's syndrome)*	1. Repeat BP 2. 24-hr Urine Catecholamines 3. Urinalysis/FBS 4. Arteriography of the renal artery 5. Lytes *(6. Serum Cortisol)*
Drug Refill 1. Substance Abuse 2. Malingering 3. Spousal Abuse 4. HIV 5. Hyperthyroidism	1. Urine Drug screen 2. Serum drug level (depending on meds) 3. HIV ELISA 4. TSH 5. EKG
Amenorrhea 1. Pregnancy 2. Menopause 3. Prolactinoma 4. Thyroid disorder 5. Anorexia nervosa	1. Genital exam 2. Serum B-HCG 3. Prolactin 4. FSH/LH 5. TSH
Vaginal Bleeding with Discharge 1. Pregnancy 2. PID 3. Endometriosis 4. UTI 5. Gonorrhea/Chlamydia	1. Serum B-HCG 2. CBC 3. C&S of discharge 4. Urinalysis 5. GC/Chlamydia by Nucleic Acid Test

Dysphagia 1. Esophageal CA 2. Achalasia 3. CREST 4. Uremia 5. Enlarged thyroid	1. Anti-centromere antibody 2. BUN/Creatinine 3. TSH 4. Esophagoscopy/Esophagogram 5. Manometry
Weakness 1. TIA 2. Myasthenia Gravis 3. Guillain-Barre 4. Multiple Sclerosis 5. Dermatomyositis	1. Carotid Doppler 2. CSF analysis 3. EMG 4. MRI 5. ESR/CK
Chest Pain 1. Acute MI 2. Pericarditis 3. Pulmonary Embolism 4. Pneumonia 5. GERD	1. CK-MB/Myoglobin/Troponin 2. ECG 3. D-dimer, V/Q scan 4. CXR 5. Manometry
Depression 1. Hypothyroidism 2. Normal Grief Reaction 3. Malignancy 4. Anemia 5. Parkinson's Disease	1. TSH/FT4/T3 2. CBC 3. CT scan of suspected area 4. AFP/CEA/PSA *(order tumor markers depending on source of malignancy)*
Sore Throat 1. Streptococcal infection 2. Infectious mononucleosis 3. Chronic Fatigue Syndrome 4. Diphtheria 5. Candidiasis	1. Rapid Strep 2. Throat GS, C&S 3. Monospot 4. CBC with diff 5. KOH Prep
Appendicitis 1. Diverticulitis 2. Gastroenteritis 3. UTI 4. PID 5. Ectopic Pregnancy	1. CBC 2. Abd U/S 3. Urinalysis 4. C&S of discharge 5. Serum B-HCG

Acute Cholecystitis 1. Hepatitis 2. PUD 3. Acute Pancreatitis 4. Colon CA 5. Pneumonia	1. HAV/HBsAg/HbcAb 2. Amylase/Lipase 3. CXR 4. Abd U/S 5. Endoscopy/Biopsy
Confusion 1. Alzheimer's Disease 2. Parkinson's Disease 3. Drug/Alcohol Intoxication 4. Hypoxia 5. Electrolyte Imbalance	1. Cranial CT 2. Alcohol Level/ Urine Drug Screen 3. Pulse Oximetry 4. ABG 5. Lytes
Blurry Vision 1. Diabetic Retinopathy 2. Hypertension 3. Glaucoma 4. Refractive Errors 5. Bacterial Conjunctivitis	1. FBS 2. Tonometry 3. Snellen's/Slit-lamp Exam 4. Repeat BP 5. Eye C&S
Insomnia 1. Hyperthyroidism 2. Generalized Anxiety Disorder 3. Obstructive Sleep Apnea 4. Depression 5. Substance Abuse	1. TSH 2. Urine Drug Screen 3. Medication level (if applicable) 4. Polysomnography 5. Lytes/CBC
Hemoptysis 1. Pulmonary TB 2. Pulmonary Embolism 3. Bronchiectasis 4. Wegener's Granulomatosis 5. Goodpasture's Syndrome	1. CXR 2. D-dimer, V/Q scan 3. Sputum C&S and stain for AFB 4. c-ANCA 5. Immunofluorescence test
Impotence 1. Psychogenic 2. Prescription Drug-induced 3. Diabetes mellitus 4. Alcoholism/Substance Abuse 5. Polymyositis	1. Stamp test 2. FBS 3. Urine Drug Screen 4. Alcohol level 5. ESR/CK

Jaundice	
1. Hepatitis	1. HbsAg/HbcAb/HAV
2. Acute Cholecystitis	2. Abdominal U/S
3. Cirrhosis	3. AFP/CA19-9
4. Hepatic CA	4. Alkaline Phosphatase
5. Pancreatic CA	5. Liver Biopsy
Leg Swelling	
1. CHF	1. ECG
2. Nephrotic Syndrome	2. 24-hr Urine Protein (24-hours)
3. Venous Insufficiency	3. UA
4. Cirrhosis	4. Doppler Ultrasound
5. Acute Post Streptococcal Nephritis	5. Liver Biopsy
Lymphadenopathy	
1. Infectious Mononucleosis	1. Monospot
2. Rubella	2. Rapid Strep
3. Hodgkin's Disease	3. Rubella Titer
4. Tuberculosis	4. CBC with diff
5. Streptococcal infection	5. PPD/CXR
Melena	
1. PUD	1. Endoscopy/Gastric Biopsy
2. Iron Ingestion	2. Serum Iron Level
3. Colon CA	3. Colonoscopy
4. Gastric CA	4. Colon biopsy
5. Crohn's Disease	5. CEA
Conjunctivitis	
1. Acute Bacterial or Viral Conjunctivitis	1. Slit lamp 2. Tonometry
2. Allergic Conjunctivitis	3. Visual Acuity Test
3. Acute Narrow Angle Glaucoma	4. Eye C&S
4. Corneal Abrasion	5. CBC
5. Contact Lens Complication	
Dysuria	
1. UTI	1. Urinalysis
2. Cystitis	2. Discharge C&S
3. PID	3. Abdominal X-ray
4. Nephrolithiasis	4. CT Scan Without Contrast
5. Malignancy (Renal or Prostate)	5. PSA

Rash	
1. Hypersensitivity Reaction	1. RAST
2. Infectious Mononucleosis	2. Monospot
3. SLE	3. ANA/anti-Smith/anti-dsDNA
4. Lyme Disease	4. Lyme Titer
5. HIV	5. HIV ELISA
Hematochezia	
1. Hemorrhoids	1. CBC/PT/PTT
2. Colon CA	2. Rectal exam
3. Ulcerative Colitis	3. Anoscopy/Sigmoidoscopy
4. Trauma	4. Colon Biopsy
5. Bleeding Disorder	5. Barium Enema
Swollen Thyroid Gland	
1. Hyperthyroidism	1. TSH
2. Hypothyroidism	2. FT4/T3
3. Multinodular goiter	3. RAI scan
4. Lymphocytic thyroiditis	4. Thyroid ultrasound
5. Thyroid CA	5. FNA
Tremors	
1. Parkinson's Disease	1. TSH
2. Essential Tremor	2. FT4/T3
3. Drug-Induced or Withdrawal Tremor	3. Serum Copper
4. Hyperthyroidism	4. Serum Ceruloplasmin/Slit Lamp
5. Wilson's Disease	5. Urine Drug Screen/Alcohol Level
(6. Electrolyte Imbalance)	*(6. Lytes)*
Claudication	
1. Deep Vein Thrombosis	1. Doppler ultrasound
2. Musculoskeletal Disease (strain or sprain)	2. Cholesterol/Triglyceride
3. Leriche's Syndrome	3. FBS/Hgb A1C
4. Arthritis	4. RF/ANA
5. Peripheral neuropathy	5. Protein C/Protein S
Premenopausal Bleeding	
1. Normal Menstrual Bleeding	1. B-HCG
2. Ovulation Bleeding	2. Pelvic Ultrasound
3. Pregnancy	3. PT/PTT
4. Blood Dyscrasia	4. Endometrial biopsy
5. Uterine Tumor	5. CBC with diff

Postmenopausal Bleeding 1. Endometrial Malignancy 2. Cervical Malignancy 3. Hormone Replacement Therapy 4. Blood Dyscrasia 5. Trauma	1. Pap Smear 2. PT/PTT 3. CBC with diff 4. Hysterocopy/Biopsy 5. Endocervical Curettage
Chronic Pelvic Pain 1. Endometriosis 2. PID 3. Adhesions 4. Tumors 5. Inflammatory Bowel Disease	1. Discharge C&S 2. Pelvic U/S 3. GC/Chlamydia by Nucleic Acid Test 4. Colonoscopy 5. Biopsy *(Endometrium or Colon)*
Dyspareunia 1. PID 2. Atrophic Vaginitis 3. Candidiasis 4. Bacterial Vaginitis/Vaginosis 5. Psychogenic	1. Discharge C & S 2. Wet mount 3. KOH prep 4. Urinalysis/C&S if indicated 5. GC/Chlamydia by Nucleic Acid Test
Hirsutism 1. Cushing's Syndrome 2. Drug-Induced 3. Polycystic Ovary Syndrome 4. Genetic Anomaly 5. Adrenal Adenoma	1. Serum Cortisol 2. Drug Level (e.g. phenytoin) 3. LH/FSH 4. Karyotyping 5. Lytes/calcium/glucose
Vertigo 1. BPPV 2. Meniere's Disease 3. Labyrinthitis 4. Acoustic neuroma 5. Drug-induced	1. Audiologic Ealuation 2. Auditory Eoked Potential 3. Caloric Stimulation 4. Electronystagmography 5. Head CT scan
Weight Loss 1. Malignancy 2. TB 3. AIDS 4. Anorexia Nervosa 5. Hyperthyroidism	1. Appropriate Tumor Marker *(e.g. AFP, HCG, PSA-depending on location)* 2. CXR 3. HIV ELISA 4. Lytes 5. TSH

Amenorrhea 1. Pregnancy 2. Pituitary tumor 3. Thyroid disorder 4. Polycystic Ovary Syndrome 5. Anorexia Nervosa	1. B-HCG 2. Prolactin level 3. TSH 4. LH/FSH 5. Lytes
Epigastric Pain 1. PUD 2. Acute MI 3. Acute Pancreatitis 4. GERD 5. Acute Cholecystitis	1. EKG/CKMB/Troponin 2. Amylase/Lipase 3. Abdominal U/S 4. FOBT 5. Endoscopy/Biopsy
RUQ Pain 1. Acute cholecystitis 2. Perforated PUD 3. Acute Pancreatitis 4. Hepatitis 5. Liver Abscess	1. Abdominal U/S 2. AXR 3. Amylase/Lipase 4. ALT/HBsAg/HBcAb 5. CBC
LUQ Pain 1. Splenic Rupture 2. Liver laceration 3. Ruptured PUD 4. Perforated Colonic CA 5. Acute Cholecystitis	1. AXR 2. Abdominal CT scan 3. CBC 4. Abdominal U/S 5. DPL (Diagnostic Peritoneal Lavage)
RLQ pain (Male) 1. Acute Appendicitis 2. Intestinal Obstruction 3. Viral Gastroenteritis 4. Perforated PUD 5. Diverticulitis	1. AXR 2. Abdominal CT scan 3. Fecal leukocyte 4. CBC with diff 5. UGIS (upper GI series)
RLQ pain (Female) 1. Acute Appendicitis 2. UTI 3. Intestinal Obstruction 4. Ectopic Pregnancy 5. Ruptured Ovarian Cyst	1. B-HCG 2. U/A 3. Abdominal U/S 4. CBC with diff 5. Pelvic Exam

LLQ pain (Male) 1. Acute Diverticulitis 2. Acute Appendicitis 3. Crohn's Disease 4. Ischemic Colitis 5. Perforated Colon CA	1. AXR 2. CBC with diff 3. FOBT 4. Abdominal CT scan 5. Colon biopsy
LLQ pain (Female) 1. Acute Diverticulitis 2. Acute Appendicitis 3. Tubo-ovarian Abscess 4. Ectopic Pregnancy 5. Ruptured Ovarian Cyst	1. B-HCG 2. FOBT 3. Abdominal U/S 4. CBC with diff. 5. Pelvic Exam
Anemia 1. Iron Deficiency 2. Lead Poisoning 3. Vitamin B12 Deficiency 4. Folate Deficiency 5. Bleeding Diathesis	1. Serum Iron/TIBC/Ferritin 2. Lead level 3. B12 level 4. Folate level 5. PT/PTT/CBC
Delirium 1. Substance Abuse 2. Drug Withdrawal 3. Delirium Tremens 4. Hypoxia 5. Electrolyte Imbalance	1. Urine Drug Screen 2. Alcohol level 3. Pulse Oximetry 4. ABG 5. Lytes
Dementia 1. Alzheimer's Disease 2. Vascular Dementia 3. Major Depression 4. Vitamin B12 Deficiency 5. Neurosyphilis/AIDS	1. MRI of the brain 2. Cholesterol/Triglyceride 3. B12 level 4. RPR/VDRL 5. HIV/ELISA
Epistaxis 1. Trauma 2. Foreign Body 3. ITP 4. Von Willebrand's Disease 5. Leukemia/Lymphoma	1. Nasal X-ray 2. CBC with diff 3. PT/PTT 4. Bleeding Time 5. Flow Cytometry

Loss of Appetite 1. Anorexia Nervosa 2. Malignancy 3. TB 4. HIV/AIDS 5. Alcoholism	1. Lytes 2. Appropriate Tumor Marker (e.g. AFP, HCG) 3. CXR 4. HIV ELISA 5. Alcohol level
Anxiety 1. Substance Abuse 2. Generalized Anxiety Disorder 3. Panic Disorder 4. Mitral Valve Prolapse 5. Hyperthyroidism	1. Urine Drug Screen 2. Echocardiography 3. TSH 4. FT4/T3 5. ECG
Neck & Shoulder Pain 1. Fracture *(humerus or clavicle)* 2. Shoulder Joint Dislocation 3. Supraspinatus Tendinitis 4. Osteoarthritis 5. Rheumatoid Arthritis	1. X-ray of Joint 2. RF 3. ESR 4. ANA 5. Synovial Fluid Analysis with C&S
Back Pain (Male) 1. Back Sprain/Strain 2. Disc Herniation 3. Osteomyelitis 4. Osteoarthritis 5. Metastatic Prostate CA	1. MRI (indicate vertebral level) 2. Lumbar X-ray 3. Urinalysis/bone scan 4. CT myelography 5. PSA
Back Pain (Female) 1. Osteoporosis 2. Disc Herniation 3. Back Sprain/Strain 4. Osteoarthritis 5. Malignancy	1. Lumbar X-ray 2. Bone Scan 3. Appropriate Tumor Marker (e.g. AFP, HCG) 4. MRI 5. CBC/ESR

Chapter 11

Work-Ups

"Sometimes I wonder whether today we take sufficient care to make a thorough physical examination before our patient starts off on the round of the laboratories, which have become so necessary that oftentimes we do not fully appreciate the value of our five senses in estimating the condition of the patient."

—William J. Mayo

- **There are five spaces for the work-ups. What if I only have four?**
- **What is the appropriate approach to ordering lab work-ups?**
- **What are the restrictions for the work-up plan?**

There are five spaces for the work-ups. What if I have only four?

This is acceptable as long as these four are all relevant to your impression or to the conditions you have listed in your differential diagnosis.

What is the appropriate approach to ordering lab work-ups?

Order the most important, most relevant and the least invasive tests first. Then order the adjunct tests next. For example, if you have a case of anemia, order a CBC first. Endoscopy or colonoscopy can follow but they should not be your priorities. Medicine is not a perfect science. Therefore, there are exceptions to the rule. The Step 2 CS is about how things are typically done in the American health care system so take each case as a typical, everyday patient encounter.

What are the restrictions for the work-up plan?

You cannot write referrals, drug treatment plans, consultations, and therapeutic procedures. You cannot order a panel of tests like comprehensive panel, hepatic function panel or iron panel. Order each test separately, like SGPT (ALT) if you want to check the liver. If you want to rule out iron deficiency anemia and you wish to do an iron panel, order iron/TIBC/ferritin on one line (note that they can be separated by a slash). The only tests allowed for ordering as a panel are: CBC, Urinalysis, Lytes, and ABG. Note that urinalysis was written as one word because, although U/A is accepted in some institutions, it can be mistaken for uric acid instead of urinalysis. To eliminate confusion, write urinalysis instead of UA or U/A. It is also recommended that you order tests from the least invasive to the most invasive. This means that if you want to rule out anemia due to GI bleed, CBC or occult blood test (OBT) must take precedence over endoscopy. Also, refrain from ordering expensive tests if you can help it.

Chapter 12

Closure

"And from the standpoint of medicine as an art for the prevention and cure of disease, the men who translate the hieroglyphics of science into the plain language of healing is certainly the more useful."
— Sir William Osler

- **How do I summarize everything?**
- **How important is the summary?**
- **How do I educate the patient?**
- **How do I handle challenging questions?**
- **What if during the two-minute discussion a patient asks me a question I can't answer?**
- **How do I deal with difficult patients?**
- **How do I deal with unexpected problems?**

How do I summarize everything?

Briefly mention the chief complaint, the most relevant portions of the history and the significant findings in the physical examination. Then give your initial impression, differential diagnosis and further work-ups you intend to do. At the end, ask the patient if she or he has any questions. Example:

I think that's all we have to do for now. Let me summarize what we have talked about. You told me that your back pain started two days ago after carrying a bag of groceries. Based on your answers to my questions and the physical examination, my initial impression of your problem is a condition called acute lumbosacral sprain I am also considering other possibilities including sciatic nerve irritation, herniated disc, osteoarthritis and prostatic carcinoma. I will be ordering some blood tests, some procedures to take pictures of your spine and a rectal exam. Do you have any question before I go?

How important is the summary?

Very important. You are given only 15 minutes to do the history, physical examination and the summary. When you summarize, you will have to tell the patient what his chief complaint was, your initial impression based on what you have gathered during the history and physical examination, and what you intend to do for further work-ups. Doing this might take about two minutes so make sure that when you are doing the physical examination, set aside the last two minutes for the summary. That means you have about five to six minutes for the interview, six to seven minutes for the PE and about two minutes for the summary.

How do I educate the patient?

This does not have to be lengthy. Patients rely on physicians not only for advice on what to do or what to take but also to give them an understanding of what their condition is. Because of time constraints in the actual exam, it may be impossible to give a patient a comprehensive discussion on the subject but you should offer two or three sentences to explain what they may be facing. Do not use medical jargon or complicated language.

How do I handle challenging questions?

Challenging questions may range from the scientific to the mundane and should be responded to with confidence and honesty. The physician must exude confidence to earn the patient's trust. And trust results in compliance. Honesty should also play a key role. If a patient asks you something you know you've seen in Robbins during your sophomore year in medical school and have already forgotten about, be forthright in saying that this is something that you are not used to seeing and are not familiar with.

Nowadays, patients can go to the internet and research their particular conditions prior to seeing a physician. Don't be caught off guard when patients come with a truckload of information. Try saying something like this, "I'm glad you did a lot of reading on the subject. It's been a while since I have encountered this and a lot has changed since then. But I will be willing to sit down with you and discuss these things when you come back for your next visit."

Examples of Challenging Questions:

For headache

Brain tumor? That sounds awfully bad!

What is a migraine?

What is temporal arteritis?

I don't think you're getting it, Doc. This doesn't appear to be that bad. But why are you ordering all these tests?

Brain tumor? Am I going to die?

For chest pain

Am I having a heart attack?

Can you do something now, please!

What is a myo…myo…something?

Quit the chit-chat. Please help me!

For abdominal pain

Is this related to pregnancy?

Is this related to the birth control pills I'm taking?

Is this related to menopause?

Is this the same illness as I had a year ago?

What if during the two-minute discussion a patient asks me a question I can't answer?

Admit that you do not know the answer to the question. Some patients in the United States are well informed regarding their conditions because of accessibility to a wide variety of resources, including the Internet. They might ask you something for which they already know the answer. Do not attempt to answer if you are unsure. Assure the patient that you will review the material and discuss the patient's questions and concerns at the patient's next appointment. Say something like this, "Mr. Jones, I'm not sure if I can give a detailed answer to your question because it has been a while since I've come across that topic. But I will refresh my knowledge about it and we can discuss your questions in detail at your next appointment."

How do I deal with difficult patients?

With calmness and compassion. SPs do this for a living and they will intentionally be rude and belligerent to see how you react and handle the situation. Thus, you have to react the way they expect you to react: calmly and compassionately. They can be rude at a certain point in the encounter, or they can be rude throughout the session; some will calm down once they hear the right words from you. Most importantly, be prepared to deal with difficult patients.

How do I deal with unexpected problems?

Maintain your cool. Always expect the unexpected. Anticipation is the name of the game and always react in a way that makes sense. For example, the patient says he wants to use the restroom and will not come out of the bathroom after several minutes. You know your clock is ticking and what will you do? Go to the restroom and ask him if he is all right. Ask him, "Is there anything I can help you with?" What if the otoscope is missing inside the room and you need to check the patient's ear? Because you are not allowed to leave the room once the exam begins, tell the patient that you will check his ears after this session. And what if after washing your hands you find there are no paper towels? Look for a clean linen (use your jacket if you can't find one) and dry your hands (of course, you do it with finesse).

Chapter 13

Patient Notes

"I wonder why you can always read a doctor's bill and you can never read his prescription."
— Finley Peter Dunne

- **How do I write the patient notes?**
- **The Step 2 CS information bulletin gives a sample of the sheet where the patient notes are written. How can I write in such a small space?**
- **Is handwriting important?**
- **What if I don't finish in the allotted time?**
- **Narrative or outline form?**
- **What if I think further work-ups are unnecessary?**

How do I write the patient notes?

Look at the samples in Part II of this book.

The Step 2 CS information bulletin gives a sample of the sheet where the patient notes are written. How can I write in such a small space?

You must know how to abbreviate. More importantly, you must know what abbreviations are accepted by the Step 2 CS. The Step 2 CS bulletin gives a partial list of acceptable abbreviations but refer to the Appendices for a complete listing. Note that certain abbreviations used in other countries are not acceptable or used in the U.S. (e.g., CLAD for cervical lymphadenopathy). Some tests like CBC and UA are acceptable and some diagnoses like DM and HIV are acceptable, too. If you are unsure if your abbreviation is acceptable, write the entire word.

Is handwriting important?

Absolutely. The physician who will grade your patient notes won't give you a point if he can't decipher your hieroglyphics. If your writing resembles "chicken scratches," spend some time improving your handwriting. Legibility is the name of the game. If it can't be read, it can't be graded.

What if I don't finish in the allotted time?

Follow the rules. Give your exam to the proctor, finished or unfinished. It is better to miss some parts than to have your entire exam invalidated because you did not follow instructions.

Narrative or outline form?

Some people find it easier to write in narrative while others prefer the outline form. Both are acceptable as long as they are legible. Others find the narrative form more time consuming and they prefer the outline form. The choice is yours.

What if I think further work-ups are unnecessary?

Enter "No studies indicated" in the space for work-ups.

Chapter 14

Travel and Visa Issues

"It is the greatest shot of adrenaline to be doing what you've wanted to do so badly. You almost feel like you could fly without the plane."
— Charles Lindberg

- **What airlines do you recommend?**
- **What hotel do you recommend?**
- **What should I do first, apply for a visa or register for the Step 2 CS?**
- **What other visa issues should I know about?**
- **What is a J-1 visa?**
- **What is an H-1B Visa?**
- **What is an O-1 visa?**

What airlines do you recommend?

Choose an airline that is not on the brink of bankruptcy to be sure that you will be able to leave on the exact date of your departure. Also, most of these airlines have cut back so much on their staffing and their service suffers as a result. Dealing with them can give you a headache and added stress, which you certainly do not want to have on the way to an examination.

What hotel do you recommend?

Depending on the test site you choose, ECFMG will recommend hotels that are in close proximity to the test site. Please refer to the official USMLE website. Look for travel information for Step 2 CS. Each evaluation center offers specific information on transportation, driving directions, parking, lodging, local hospital, emergency telephone numbers, and other travel resources. It also lists the respective city's Visitor's Bureau website and telephone numbers.

What should I do first, apply for a visa or register for the Step 2 CS?

After you have passed USMLE Step 1, apply for a visa immediately. You must obtain a visa before you apply for the Step 2 CS because if you register for the Step 2 CS first and your visa is denied, you lose the $1,200 you paid for the exam. If the consulate in your country requires you to register for the exam, you have no choice and you must register first before you can apply for a visa. Ask friends from your own country who have been through the process. They are your best resource of information because visa policies can vary from country to country, especially now during the post 9/11 era.

What other visa issues should I know about?

When you apply for a visa to take the USMLE CS in the United States, you will have to apply as a tourist. U. S. policies continue to change since September 11, 2001 and the best way to keep updated is to go to the BCIS (formerly, INS) website. Obtaining a visa from countries with large Muslim populations can be a difficult because of certain issues regarding terrorism, but this should not discourage you. It can be difficult but it is not impossible.

When you apply for a tourist visa, you must have a valid reason why you want to enter the United States. Taking the USMLE CS is a valid reason because it is not offered anywhere else outside the continental United States. In order for you to have a USMLE document to show the consulate in your country, you must have applied and paid USMLE. This means that you will have to pay $1,200 with no guarantee that you will be granted a visa to take the exam in the United States. Most consuls look at each application on an individual basis and what holds true for others may not hold true for you, and vice versa. It's worth the effort.

What is a J-1 visa?

For those who have passed the required USMLE steps and are seeking residency training, the issue is a bit different. You can either apply for a J-1 visa, which is a "training" visa, or an H-1B visa which is a "working" visa.

The J-1 visa is a non-immigrant visa issued by the U.S. consulate to an applicant seeking a residency or fellowship training in the United States. The visa is valid for seven years but the bearer of the visa is obliged to return to his or her home country for at least two years before he/she can return to the United States. Form DS 2019 is issued by the Educational Commission for Foreign Medical Graduates (ECFMG) upon completion of the required examinations. This document basically informs the U.S. consulate in your home country that you are eligible to enter the United States. You will also be required to obtain a signed document from your country's health department certifying the need for trained physicians in your chosen field of specialty. It will then be up to the U.S. consulate to decide if your J-1 visa will be approved.

There is a saying that goes, "Once a J-1, always a J-1." This is because most J-1 visa holders often encounter difficulties converting their visas into another visa form which becomes important when you are nearing the end of your residency or fellowship training. With a J-1, you cannot stay in the U.S. after your training is completed, even if you have been in the U.S. for fewer than seven years. You also cannot work as an attending physician because of your status.

One way of prolonging your stay in the U.S. is by getting a "waiver" which permits a non-immigrant to stay after the training period as long as he agrees to practice in an area designated by the Department of Agriculture as "underserved." A significant number of foreign doctors vie for these spots and the competition can be fierce. However, once you have obtained a waiver, you will be on your way to obtaining an H-1B visa which allows you to work legally in the United States. An H-1B can be further converted into a "green card" or permanent residence status.

What is an H-1B Visa?

This is a better visa than a J-1 because you do not have to return to your native country for at least two years before being allowed back into the United States. There are several requirements that must be fulfilled before this visa is approved, including:

1. ECFMG certification (which means that you must have passed USMLE step 1, Step 2 CK and Step 2 CS)
2. Pass USMLE Step 3.
3. Must have a license in the particular state where you intend to do your residency.

Not all residency programs sponsor an H-1B visa, although most sponsor a J-1 visa. That is why it is important to know what visa your prospective residency program is willing to support. There are several websites that offer information on these but you will have to pay for the information. Included in the Appendices of this book is a partial list of hospitals considered IMG-friendly because they have historically sponsored either a J-1, an H-1B or both. If you do not have this information, be sure to ask about this issue during your interview.

It may take 2–3 months to process your H-1B application; be sure to take this into consideration. The process can be expedited to 14 days but it costs about $1,000 more to do this and some residency programs may not be willing to absorb this expense on your behalf.

It is important to know that residency interviews usually take place during the months from October to January. The match takes place in March and residencies begin in July. Make sure you have sufficient time if you are considering applying for an H-1B visa.

What is an O-1 visa?

O-1 is a visa given to foreigners who have proven themselves outstanding in their particular field through publications in major journals, awards, and recognized accomplishments. For IMGs, this is often a last resort at the end of a residency (if they qualify) when their J-1 visa is about to expire and they are unable to obtain a waiver for an extension of their current visa.

Chapter 15

Exam Day

"Needless fear and panic over disease or misfortune that seldom materialize are simply bad habits. By proper ventilation and illumination of the mind it is possible to cultivate tolerance, poise and real courage."
— Elie Metchnikoff

- **Can I go to the building the day before the exam?**
- **How important is a good night's sleep before the exam?**
- **Any advice for controlling my anxiety?**
- **What if I forget my official permit on the day of the exam?**
- **Can I talk in our native language to my friend who is also taking the exam?**
- **After the exam, can I discuss my case with other Step 2 CS candidates?**
- **Can I bring a friend or a relative with me inside the building?**
- **What should I wear in the exam?**
- **Can I wear a wristwatch?**
- **How about cellphones and pagers?**
- **Can I wear perfume or cologne during the exam?**
- **Can I bring mints? Can I chew gum?**
- **Do I have to bring my own lunch or dinner?**
- **Can I bring my luggage to the test site?**
- **Will there be an orientation before the exam?**
- **What else do I have to bring, aside from the white coat?**
- **How important is patient information on the door?**

- **How many patients will I have?**
- **How long will the exams last?**
- **What do I need to do after the exam?**
- **Who will evaluate my performance?**
- **What do you suggest I do while waiting for the results?**
- **I flunked the Step 2 CS. Any suggestions?**
- **Should I start working on my residency application while waiting for the result?**
- **Can you name some hospitals or institutions that traditionally accept IMGs in their residency programs?**

THE DAY BEFORE THE EXAM

Can I go to the building the day before the exam?

You cannot enter the building unless you are taking the exam on that day. It is a good idea to drive by and see where the building and the parking lot are located so you won't be searching for them on exam day.

How important is a good night's sleep before the exam?

Extremely important. Be ready for unforeseen, unrelated problems to crop up right before the big day. You must be able to put a lid on your emotions so you can snooze the night away on the eve of the exam.

Any advice for controlling my anxiety?

Psyche yourself up and remember the following two rules. The first rule is to always think of the exam as another day's work. The second rule is, always remember rule one.

ON THE DAY OF THE EXAM

What if I forget my official permit on the day of the exam?

You have to call the Step 2 CS office to verify this matter because policies change. Best advice: tie a string on your index finger to remind you to bring your permit to the exam.

Can I talk in our native language to my friend who is also taking the exam?

Try not to. It is impolite, and it is forbidden once the exam has begun.

After the exam, can I discuss my case with other Step 2 CS candidates?

Absolutely not. Never discuss your case; Not during or even after the exam, and not during the break. Discussing your case with other candidates is equivalent to cheating and USMLE doesn't tolerate this. It is also important that you speak English all the time. As long as you are within the building premises, even if you are talking to a friend who shares the same language with you, always speak in English. This is a fair way of assuring the integrity of the exam.

Can I bring a friend or a relative with me inside the building?

No. You will only be allowed to enter the building if you have a Step 2 CS permit, which will be provided to you once you register for the exam. Your friend or relative can wait for you outside, or better yet, in the hotel since there is no comfortable waiting area outside the ECFMG building.

What should I wear in the exam?

Wear comfortable but professional attire. In the U.S., professional attire for male physician consists of a white jacket over a long-sleeved shirt with a necktie. Pants should be formal to semi-formal and shoes are preferably leather. You have to bring your own jacket and it can be plain white or you can bring one with your name or your institution's name embroidered on it. A matching coat and tie would be too much because you will end up removing the coat so you can put the white jacket on. Never wear jeans: this is considered unprofessional in the United States even if wearing Levi's is a status symbol in your country. A pair of scrubs and sneakers can also be worn under the white gown if this is your preference. Female physicians can wear a coordinated blouse and skirt or any semi-formal dress that won't show too much cleavage or too much thigh. Wear comfortable shoes. In other words, wear something you would wear in church.

Can I wear a wristwatch?

You can wear an analog wristwatch but not a digital one. Do not look at your watch too often during the interview or while doing the physical exam because the patient may think you are in a hurry and paying more attention to the time than to his welfare.

How about cell phones and pagers?

Cell phones, pagers, PDAs, cameras, digital watches, or any two-way communication devices are not allowed within the building premises.

Can I wear perfume or cologne during the exam?

A lot of hospitals in the United States do not allow clinicians who have direct contact with patients to wear colognes or perfumes because of possible allergic reactions from patients. What may smell like roses to you may be smell like a dead rodent to another. Play it safe — and don't wear scent during the exam (but be sure to take care of the basics — deodorant and mouthwash).

Can I bring mints? Can I chew gum?

You can bring mints and gums before the exam, but the contents of your pockets will be placed in a certain area before you begin the exam.

Do I have to bring my own lunch or dinner?

Food will be provided during the break so you do not have to bring your own. There will be two breaks — a 30-minute break and a 15-minute break — during which food or refreshments will be served.

Can I bring my luggage to the test site?

You will be provided with a small space on a shelf where your wallet, purse, passport or other things you brought with you can be kept while you take the exam. A small luggage can probably fit in there but not a big one. To be sure, just check out of the hotel after you complete the exam so you won't have to worry where to put your luggage. If you do not want to pay an extra day for the hotel, inquire with your specific CS evaluation center and ask them if you can bring your luggage.

Will there be an orientation before the exam?

Yes. The USMLE Step 2 CS online bulletin states that a short orientation and demonstration will be given to cover the diagnostic instruments you can expect to see in the rooms and other important information regarding the exam. During this period, ask any questions you have. The Step 2 CS staff is very friendly and helpful and they make every effort to make the process a little less tense.

What else do I have to bring, aside from the white coat?

Bring two forms of photo identification (driver's license and passport), a stethoscope, an analog watch and your permit for the exam. If you don't have a driver's license, bring another government-issued or institution-issued photo ID in addition to the passport. They also do not allow any digital watches so if you think you will need a wristwatch, bring an analog one. Remember, quick glances at your watch. Don't make the patient feel that your time is more important than their illness. Some suggest placing the face of your wristwatch on the palmar aspect of your wrist so you can make quick glances without the patient noticing it. Most importantly, bring your permit.

How important is patient information on the door?

This information is critical. This informtion — the patient's name, age, chief complaint and vital signs — will determine how you will proceed with your data gathering and physical examination. Watch the Step 2 CS online video to see what this doorway information will look like. Although Step 2 CS fairly posts this same information inside the room, it would save you time if you write it while outside the room as you gather your thoughts and decide on what actions to take for that particular encounter.

How many patients will I have?

Step 2 CS gives each examinee 11 to 12 patients. The number is a lot less important than the quality of service you are expected to render. Treat each patient as a human being and not merely a case number. The most important thing to remember is that we are dealing with life and a patient can be somebody's mother or somebody's father. As physicians, we need to act with courtesy, care and compassion in all instances because those are what distinguish our profession from others.

How long will the exams last?

It will take about eight hours or less for the entire exam. This timeframe includes two breaks (a 30-minute and a 15-minute break) during which food will be provided.

AFTER THE EXAM

What do I need to do after the exam?

Relax and see the city.

Who will evaluate my performance?

You will be evaluated by the SPs and by physician examiners. The SPs will evaluate the communication, data gathering and thoroughness of your physical examination. A physician examiner will evaluate your patient notes. Your performance inside the room is recorded on video cameras so the physician examiner can access it. Just pretend that somebody is watching you all the time so do everything within the bounds of reason and medical ethics. But don't let this scare you. If you act and think as the doctor you were trained to be, you should do well.

What do you suggest I do while waiting for the results?

Pray.

I flunked the Step 2 CS. Any suggestions?

Step 2 CS is not only a gauge of your history taking and physical examination skills. It is also a yardstick for politeness, ethics, decision-making skills, rapport, likeability and common sense. Many physicians, especially those who come from other countries display professional superiority when dealing with typical patients because they are used to being treated like demigods in their own countries. This attitude is not well received in the United States. If you failed the first time, apply for an observership in a U.S. institution so you can get a glimpse of how things work here. Or read books and watch videos on how to do the interview process the American way.

Should I start working on my residency application while waiting for the result?

It depends on when you intend to start residency. Your timing strategy must be based on the residency application "timelines." Interviews usually start in October and end in January; some, but not many, programs conduct interviews until February. Match date is mid-March. Scramble is usually the day after the match day and post-match starts thereafter until the start of residency which is July.

Some programs will grant you interviews even without results from the Step 2 CS if you explain you have taken the exam and are waiting for the result.

Can you name some hospitals or institutions that traditionally accept IMGs in their residency programs?

Refer to the Appendices at the end of this book for a list of traditionally IMG-friendly hospitals.

Part II:
Mock Exam

IMPORTANT POINTERS ON PERFORMING THE MOCK EXAMS

- Each case presented here consists of a case presentation, interview questions and patient notes.
- The most effective way to practice is with a study partner. Reverse roles after each case.
- If no medical study partner is available, ask a friend, spouse or relative to act as a patient.
- Use a timer and set it as directed in the Step 2 CS bulletin (presently 15 minutes for the interview and physical examination and 10 minutes for patient notes).
- Copy each case presentation page, cut it out from the questionnaire and randomly post it on the door where you are going to do the mock exam.
- Ask the study partner to check off the list of interview questions you ask. Ask your partner to note which ones you miss.
- The case presentation format presented here may not reflect the same format as the actual exam. The format presented in these mock exams should be used as a guide to point out where you should start focusing your line of questioning.
- Note that on the interview questions for cases involving pain, you will see that you can use a generic format for a systematic interview by following the mnemonic "LMNOPQRST" which corresponds to the list below:

  L – ocation
  M – edication
  N – nausea, vomiting, fever (NVF)
  O – nset
  P – recipitating/Palliating
  Q – uality
  R – adiation/Relieving Factors
  S – everity (scale of 1–10)
  T – iming
- Always include the chief complaint.
- The HPI questions can vary but the questions for past medical history, family history, social history and sexual history can have a generic format.
- If the patient is a female, always include an OB/GYN history. If pressed for time, note the OB score at minimum.
- Aside from the main interview, there are three things that should be included: the introduction, the transition statement from the interview to the physical exam, and the closing statements.
- Always anticipate that each patient will ask a challenging question.
- Wash your hands before and after the physical exam.
- DO NOT repeat any painful maneuvers.
- When examining joint pains, also check the joint above it, below it and on the contralateral side.
- Write the patient note as legibly as possible as if it is the actual exam.
- Study Case No.1 and the subsequent analysis of each part to understand how the mock exams were set up.

CASE NO. 1

Mrs. Betty Smith is a 52-year-old white female who came to the clinic with headaches.

Vital Signs:

T 101.4° F

P 100

R 20

BP 130/85

EXPECTED TASKS

1. Gather the necessary clinical information.
2. Perform a focused and pertinent physical examination.
3. Discuss your diagnostic impressions and differential diagnosis with the patient.
4. Discuss work-ups to be ordered.
5. Complete the patient note after seeing the patient.

Headache

(Knocks on door. Do not turn the lights on if the room is dim. Ask patient first. You might be dealing with photophobia of meningitis.)

Hi, I'm Dr. _______ and I'm here to examine you today. Do you prefer to be called Mrs. Smith or Betty?

☐ 1. What brings you in today?
(Mnemonic: LMNOPQRST)
Location: Where exactly do you feel the pain?
Medications: Are you taking any medication right now?
Nausea and vomiting, fever, weakness? Other symptoms?
Onset: When did this start?
Precipitating Factor/**P**rodrome: What makes it worse? Do you feel any warning signs before the pain starts?
Quality: How would you describe the pain?
Radiation/**R**elieving Factors: Does it go anywhere? What makes it go away?
Severity: On a scale of 1–10, where 10 is the most painful, at what level would you rank your pain?
Timing: At what time does it usually occur? How often?

☐ 2. Have you had any fever recently? *(R/O meningitis)*

☐ 3. Any history of head trauma? How about sinusitis? Hypertension?

☐ 4. Any changes in your vision? *(R/O temporal arteritis.)* How about tearing with nasal discharge? *(R/O cluster headache.)*

☐ 5. Have you ever been hospitalized before? Any accidents or injuries? Allergies? Any similar episodes of headaches before?

- ☐ 6. Are your parents living? How's their health? How about your brothers and sisters? Do you have children? How's their health?
- ☐ 7. What is your occupation? Do you feel stressed at work? Do you use tobacco products? How about alcohol? Do you take any kind of recreational drugs? Who do you live with?
- ☐ 8. I will be asking some questions of a sensitive nature that will help me better assess your total health. I can assure you that this will all be kept confidential. Is that okay with you? Are you sexually active? Do you have sex with the same sex, opposite sex or both? Do you use any protective barrier? How would you describe your sexual life — good or bad? Why is that?

Thanks for answering these questions. Now I will be examining some parts of your body but let me wash my hands first. *(Wash hands.)*

- ☐ 9. I will be shining this light into your eyes, just look straight ahead. *(meningitis has photophobia)*
- ☐ 10. I will be checking your eyes with this instrument. Just look straight ahead. *(Use ophthalmoscope. Check for hypertensive retinopathy signs.)*
- ☐ 11. I will now feel and tap your sinuses. Let me know if you feel any pain, OK?
- ☐ 12. Now, let me feel the blood vessels in your temple. Let me know if you feel any pain when I touch it.
- ☐ 13. I'm going to check your neck for stiffness. I'll try to make your chin touch your chest, Ok? *(Brudzinski's sign)*
- ☐ 14. I'll now try to fold your knee and straighten it. *(Kernig's sign)*
- ☐ 15. I'll test your muscle strength now. Raise your arms/forearms/hand against my hand. Now let's do it downward.
- ☐ 16. Now raise your thigh/leg/feet against my strength. Now, let's do it downward.
- ☐ 17. Let's check your reflexes now. *(Do biceps, triceps, knee and Achilles.)*

Now let me summarize what you've told me. You said your headache is located in __________. My initial impression of your condition is meningitis. But I am also considering other possibilities like migraine headache, cluster headache, and sinusitis. Also, in cases like this, we also want to make sure that we are not dealing with a brain tumor, so I am ordering some blood tests and a CT scan of the head. Do you have any questions?

Challenging Questions:

Brain tumor? That sounds awfully bad!
What is a migraine?
What is a cluster headache?
I don't think you're getting it, Doc. This doesn't appear to be that bad. Why are you ordering all these tests?
Brain tumor? Am I going to die?
How did I get this?

History:

cc:	headache
HPI:	52 y/o female c/o headache on the L side of her frontal and parietal areas. Described as dull, continuous, non-radiating and occurring upon waking up in the morning. Not relieved by Tylenol but slightly relieved by rest. There is an associated high fever but no nausea or vomiting. Photophobia is present since the onset of headache 2 days ago but no aura or scotoma. Severity is 9/10 on the pain scale.
PMH:	hospitalized 3 yrs ago for food poisoning.
FamH:	father in nursing home with hypertension; mother's history unknown
SocH:	works as a librarian; not under stress
SexH:	sex with husband only.
OB/GynH:	G2P2, postmenopausal.

Physical Examination:

Gen:	A&O X3 but in acute pain
VS:	T: 101.4° F BP: 130/85
Eyes:	PERRLA with photophobia, normal funduscopic findings, normal visual acuity using the Snellen chart; no conjunctival injection
Sinus:	no tenderness on palpation or percussion
Neuro:	Brudzinski's sign (+), Kernig's sign (+) CN III-XII intact Motor strength: 5/5 X4 extremities Sensation: intact DTRs: ++

Differential Diagnosis:

1. Meningitis
2. Migraine Headache
3. Intracranial Tumor
4. Cluster Headache
5. Sinusitis

Diagnostic Work-ups:

1. CSF analysis and C&S
2. CT scan of the head
3. CBC with diff
4. ESR
5. X-ray of sinuses

Now the analysis of each part.

Mrs. Betty Smith is a 52-year-old white female who came to the clinic because of headaches.

This is important information that will determine how you will proceed with your questioning. The name can be given as a full name or just the last name. The age and gender will be given but the ethnicity or race can be included or not. Then the chief complaint is given at the end, which should make you focus on the kinds of questions you will ask and the physical exams you will perform. But remember, some patients will tell you their main complaint but after doing the interview and performing the physical exam, your impression of the chief complaint can change considerably.

Vital Signs:

T 101.4° F
P 100
R 20
BP 130/85

The vital signs will give you clues as to what condition you will have to deal with. If the patient has a fever, you may be dealing with an infectious, inflammatory or neoplastic condition. An increased pulse rate or a high BP should tip you off that you have to focus on the cardiovascular system. Likewise, an abnormal respiratory rate should steer you into a pulmonary or cardiac pathology.

EXPECTED TASKS

1. Gather the necessary clinical information.
2. Perform a focused and pertinent physical examination.
3. Discuss your diagnostic impressions and differential diagnosis with the patient.
4. Discuss work-ups to be ordered.
5. Complete the patient note after seeing the patient.

This is simply a list of direction on what you are expected to do during this patient encounter.

Hi, I'm Dr. _______ and I'm here to examine you today. Do you prefer to be called Mrs. Smith or Betty?

This is the introduction. You have to tell the patient who you are and what you are there for. You can also ask the patient how she wants to be addressed because this is your first step in establishing rapport with the patient. Do not hesitate to call patients by their first names if that is what they prefer because in the United States, you can call people by their first name even if they are a lot older than you. However, how patients are addressed can vary by region. In some parts of the U.S., addressing a patient by first name and/or by an incorrect salutation (Ms. or Mrs.), would be considered impolite.

☐ **1. What brings you in today?**

This is asking the patient their chief complaint. Although it was already printed on the paper before you enter the room, asking the patient this question will confirm what the patient came in for. Put a check here if your study partner asked this question.

Location: Where do you feel the pain, exactly?
Medications: Are you taking any medication right now?
Nausea and Vomiting, Weakness? Other symptoms?
Onset: When did this start?
Precipitating Factor /Prodrome: What makes it worse? Do you feel any warning before the pain starts?
Quality: How would you describe the pain?
Radiation/Relieving Factors: Does it go anywhere? What makes it go away?
Severity: On a scale of 1–10, where 10 is the most painful, at what level would you rank your pain?
Timing: At what time does it usually occur? How often?

These are the questions that will determine what you will write on the History of Present Illness (HPI). This can vary from one case to another. This is also the part where you do a focused review of systems. Again, the questions you ask should be relevant to the issue you are dealing with.

You might notice that in some cases you can create a mnemonic so the organization and fluidity of your interview will impress the SP. For example, any case presenting with pain, the traditional mnemonic OPQRST (onset, precipitating, quality, radiation, severity, timing) can work. But I have added LMN (location, medications taken, nausea and other symptoms like vomiting, fever, etc.) which makes it more complete. Create your own mnemonics if you prefer. Below are a few examples of mnemonics I have used successfully:

PPP DIABETIC (see Case No.15) if you suspect Diabetes mellitus
MNOPQRST (see Case No. 20) for hearing loss

Practice writing the mnemonic on a clean sheet of paper before you start interviewing your study partner so you won't miss anything.

☐ **2. Have you had any fever recently? *(R/O meningitis.)***
☐ **3. Any history of head trauma? How about sinusitis? Hypertension?**
☐ **4. Any changes in your vision? *(R/O temporal arteritis.)* How about tearing with nasal discharge? *(R/O cluster headache.)***

Additional questions to rule out other conditions and narrow down the differential diagnosis.

☐ **5. Have you ever been hospitalized before? Any accidents or injuries? Allergies? Any similar episodes of headaches before?**
☐ **6. Are your parents living? How's their health? How about your brothers and sisters? Do you have children? How's their health?**

- ☐ **7. What is your occupation? Do you feel stressed at work? Do you use tobacco products? How about alcohol? Do you take any kind of recreational drugs? Who do you live with?**
- ☐ **8. I will be asking some questions of a sensitive nature that will help me better assess your total health. I can assure you that this will all be kept confidential. Is that okay with you? Are you sexually active? Do you have sex with the same sex, opposite sex or both? Do you use any protective barrier? How would you describe your sexual life — good or bad? Why is that?**

I call this part the "mainstay" of the interview process because these questions should always be a permanent part of the interview. This include the past medical history (PMH), family history (FH or FamH), social history (SH or SocH), sexual history (SexH or SxH), OB/GYN history and Developmental History (if applicable). These questions can be asked in many different ways but for the purpose of the exam, adhere to the script you have been practicing all along. In addition, you can also use this portion as a "fall-back" script in the event you become overanxious. For sexual issues, carefully select the questions appropriate for the case.

Thanks for answering these questions. Now I will be examining some parts of your body but let me wash my hands first. *(Wash hands.)* Let me put this drape on so you'll feel more comfortable. *(Drape patient.)*

I refer to this as the transition zone. As a pathologist in training, missing the transition zone can mean the difference between a lawsuit and a paycheck. Same is true with Step 2 CS — missing it can mean the difference between passing and failing. This portion has three important components:

1. *Let the patient know that you are finished with the interview and now ready to do the physical examination.*
2. *Letting the patient know and emphasizing that you are washing your hands — which, by the way, if missed, can certainly cost you points!*
3. *Offering to drape the patient which will add points to your being respectful of his privacy and comfort.*

- ☐ **9. I will be shining this light into your eyes, just look straight ahead. (meningitis has photophobia)**
- ☐ **10. Now, I will be checking your eyes with this instrument. Just look straight ahead. (Use ophthalmoscope. Check for hypertensive retinopathy signs.)**
- ☐ **11. I will now feel and tap your sinuses. Let me know if you feel any pain, OK?**
- ☐ **12. Now, let me feel the blood vessels in your temple. Let me know if you feel any pain when I touch it.**
- ☐ **13. I'm going to check your neck for stiffness. I'll try to make your chin touch your chest, Ok? (Brudzinski's sign)**
- ☐ **14. I'll now try to fold your knee and straighten it. (Kernig's sign)**
- ☐ **15. I'll test your muscle strength now. Raise your arms/forearms/hand against my hand. Now let's do it downward.**

☐ **16. Now raise your thigh/leg/feet against my strength. Now, let's do it downward.**
☐ **17. Let's check your reflexes now. (Do biceps, triceps, knee and Achilles.)**

Always remember to tell the patient ahead of time what you are going to do in the physical examination. This will help to make the patient more cooperative and will also make him confident that you know what you are doing. If the maneuver is going to be painful, you may want to alert him to that possibility. NEVER repeat any painful maneuver.

Now let me summarize what you've told me. You said your headache is located in _________. My initial impression of your condition is meningitis. But I am also considering other possibilities like migraine headache, cluster headache, and sinusitis. Also, in cases like this, we want to make sure that we are not dealing with a brain tumor, so I am ordering some blood tests and a CT scan of the head. Do you have any questions?

In the Summary, tell the patient that you are finished and briefly discuss the chief complaint and the significant findings in the interview and physical examination. Then give your initial impression and what further tests you will be ordering. If you are running out of time and you are still doing the PE and you only have a few minutes left, try to squeeze the summary in because it constitutes a significant portion of the interview score. It is always helpful to memorize and get used to a generic summary so you won't be lost for words during the crucial last few minutes of the encounter.

Possible challenging questions for headache

Brain tumor? That sounds awfully bad!
What is a migraine?
What is a cluster headache?
I don't think you're getting it, Doc. This doesn't appear to be that bad. But why are you ordering all these tests?
Brain tumor? Am I going to die?

Always expect a question from the patient.

*Now the **Patient Notes**...*

History:

cc:	headache
HPI:	52 y/o female c/o headache on the L side of her frontal and parietal areas. Described as dull, continuous, non-radiating and occurring upon waking up in the morning. Not relieved by Tylenol but slightly relieved by rest. There is an associated high fever but no nausea or vomiting. Photophobia is present since the onset of headache 2 days ago but no aura or scotoma. Severity is 9/10 on the pain scale.

PMH:	hospitalized 3 yrs ago for food poisoning.
FamH:	father in nursing home with hypertension; mother's history unknown.
SocH:	works as a librarian; not under stress.
SexH:	sex with husband only.
OB/GynH:	G2P2, postmenopausal.

In the history, always write the chief complaint (cc) on the patient notes. The HPI can be in an outline format or a narrative format. For the sake of consistency, use only one format.

In writing the rest of the history (PMH, FH, SocH, SexH), knowing the accepted abbreviations helps. For example, writing "cig (–)" is faster than writing "non-smoker" or "does not smoke"; writing etoh (–) is a shorter way of writing "does not drink alcoholic beverages."

If the patient is a woman, do not forget the OB score. If dealing with a pediatric case, always remember to include the developmental milestones.

Physical Examination:

Gen:	A&O X3 but in acute pain
VS:	T: 101.4° F BP: 130/85
Eyes:	PERRLA with photophobia, normal fundoscopic findings, normal visual acuity using the Snellen chart; no conjunctival injection
Sinus:	no tenderness on palpation or percussion
Neuro:	Brudzinski's sign (+), Kernig's sign (+) CN III-XII intact Motor strength: 5/5 X4 extremities Sensation: intact DTRs: ++

Writing the physical examination results should include only the pertinent ones. Your performance of the physical examination will be graded by the SP. The patient notes will be graded by a physician. Although graded by two different persons, write only the physical examination results that you have performed. The entire session is video taped and can be reviewed if there is a question or discrepancy between what was performed and what was written.

Differential Diagnosis:

1. **Meningitis**
2. **Migraine Headache**
3. **Intracranial Tumor**
4. **Cluster Headache**
5. **Sinusitis**

This section has five numbers where you list your initial impression or differential diagnosis. Place your main initial impression in number 1 and the rest of your differentials in the succeeding numbers. If you only fill up to 4, that is OK. To be on the safe side, offer 5 whenever possible. Certain situations will only have 1 or 2 in the the differentials but this doesn't happen often. Be prepared if it does.

Diagnostic Work-ups:

1. **CSF analysis and C&S**
2. **CT scan of the head**
3. **CBC with diff**
4. **ESR**
5. **X-ray of sinuses**

This section must be consistent with the conditions you have enumerated in the differential diagnosis. The numbers do not necessarily have to correspond but make sure they are all relevant. For example, if you put hyperthyroidism as your Number 1 differential diagnosis, you can put TSH in number 1 and thyroid scan in number 2 under work-ups. You can also combine several tests together in one number (usually, if they can be taken out of the same specimen) and separate them with a forward slash (/) like writing TSH/FT4/T3 in number 1. If you only have 3 or 4 work-ups instead of 5, that will be acceptable if they are pertinent to what you have written in the differential diagnosis.

Moreover, because the actual exam places restrictions and disallows performance of some physical examinations including breast exams, genital exams (internal or external), and rectal exams, you should list these exams as part of your work-up if deemed necessary.

CASE NO. 2

Mr. Gerald Chen is a 60-year-old male who came in with chest pain.

Vital Signs:

T 99.8°F
P 110
R 22
BP 130/80

EXPECTED TASKS

1. Gather the necessary clinical information.
2. Perform a focused and pertinent physical examination.
3. Discuss your diagnostic impressions and differential diagnosis with the patient.
4. Discuss work-ups to be ordered.
5. Complete the patient note after seeing the patient.

Chest Pain

(Knocks)

Hi, I'm Dr. ______. How are you today? *(Shakes patient's hand.)* I'm here to examine you and ask you a few questions. By the way, do you prefer to be called Gerald or Mr. Chen?

- ☐ 1. So, what brings you in today?
  (Mnemonics: LMNOPQRST)
- ☐ 2. **L**ocation: Can you show me exactly where the pain is?
- ☐ 3. **M**edications: Are you taking any medications? Have you taken any recently?
- ☐ 4. **N** & V: Do you have any nausea? Vomiting? Weakness?
- ☐ 5. **O**nset: When did it start?
- ☐ 6. **P**recipitating/**P**alliating: What makes it worse? What makes it better?
- ☐ 7. **Q**uality: How would you describe the pain?
- ☐ 8. **R**adiation: Does the pain spread?
- ☐ 9. **S**everity: On a scale of 1–10, where 10 is the most painful, where would you rate this pain?
- ☐ 10. **T**iming: Does it occur at a particular time of day?
- ☐ 11. Does the pain occur when you overeat? Do antacids relieve it? *(R/O GERD.)*
- ☐ 12. Do you feel a sharp pain on your chest when you breathe? *(R/O costochondritis.)*
- ☐ 13. Have you had any illnesses in the past? Any accidents or allergies?
- ☐ 14. I will be asking you about diseases in the family, OK? Are your parents healthy? How about your brothers and sisters? How about your wife and children? Any history of diabetes or heart attack in the family?
- ☐ 15. What kind of work do you do? Do you smoke? Drink? Do you exercise? Do you use any recreational drugs?

☐ 16. Now, I will be asking you some questions of a sensitive nature. I can assure you that anything you say will be kept confidential. I just need to ask these questions so I can have a clearer picture of your overall health. Are you sexually active? Are your partners men, women or both? How many partners have you had during the past year? Do you use condoms?

Thanks for answering all these questions. At this point, I will be doing a physical examination but let me wash my hands first. *(Wash hands.)* Would you be more comfortable if I put this drape on your legs? *(Drape patient if he answers yes.)*

☐ 17. I would like to listen to your heart and feel your heartbeat.
☐ 18. Just breathe normally while I gently press on your ribs.
☐ 19. Can you say "99" while I move my hands on various areas of your chest and back? *(Fremitus)*
☐ 20. I will be tapping your back.
☐ 21. I will be listening to your lungs. Breathe in and breathe out.

Now let me summarize what we have talked about. You came in because of chest pain. Based on the history and the physical examination my initial impression of your condition is _______. I am also considering other possibilities so I will be ordering some tests to make sure that we consider all the possible scenarios so we can make better decisions on how we will deal with your condition. Do you have any questions before I go?

Challenging Questions:

Am I having a heart attack?
Can you do something now, please!
What is a myo...myo...something?
Quit the chit-chat. Please help me!
What is troponin?
What causes this?

Chest Pain

History:

cc:	chest pain
HPI:	60 y/o Asian male business executive c/o chest pain that started 3 hours ago and characterized as chest tightness radiating to the shoulders, jaw and back. The pain occurs both at rest and during exertion. Graded as 8/10 on the pain scale. He has been taking aspirin and metoprolol daily since his "mild heart attack" was diagnosed 2 yrs. ago.
PMH:	hospitalization for heart attack 2 yrs. ago, no other similar episode since then; no allergies, no accidents, no h/o surgery
FH:	mother has HTN, father died of a heart attack at age 50
SocH:	cig(+) 1 ppd X 10 yrs; etoh only in social gatherings; illicit drug use (–).
ROS:	(+) chest tightness, no fever, no nausea, no vomiting, no syncope

Physical Examination:

Gen:	A&O, in acute pain and distress
VS:	BP: 130/80 T: 99.8° F HR:110 RR: 22 cpm
CV:	NRRR, PMI not displaced; no murmurs, gallops, rubs or clicks
Lungs:	symmetrical; N breath sounds B/L, no rales, no dullness, normal vocal and tactile fremitus
Musculoskeletal:	No point tenderness on the anterior and posterior chest areas

Differential Diagnosis:

1. Acute MI
2. Angina
3. Pericarditis
4. Pulmonary Embolism
5. Costochondritis

Diagnostic Work-ups:

1. EKG
2. Troponin/Myoglobin/CK-MB
3. CXR
4. PFT
5. Pulse oximetry

CASE NO. 3

Mrs. Linda Holloway is a 42-year-old female who came in with abdominal pain.

Vital Signs:

T 99.9° F
P 70
R 14
BP 125/85

EXPECTED TASKS

1. Gather the necessary clinical information.
2. Perform a focused and pertinent physical examination.
3. Discuss your diagnostic impressions and differential diagnosis with the patient.
4. Discuss work-ups to be ordered.
5. Complete the patient note after seeing the patient.

Abdominal Pain (Acute Cholecystitis)

(Knocks)

Hi, I'm Dr. ______ and I'm here to examine you today. Do you prefer to be called Mrs. Holloway or Linda?

☐ 1. So, what brings you in today?
(Mnemonic: LMNOPQRST)
Location: Can you point with one finger exactly where the pain is?
Medications: Are you taking any medication right now?
Nausea and vomiting, weakness? Other symptoms?
Onset: When did this start?
Precipitating Factor: What makes it worse?
Quality: How would you describe the pain?
Radiation/**R**elieving Factors: Does it go anywhere? What makes it go away?
Severity: On a scale of 1–10, where 10 is the most painful, at what level would you rank your pain?
Timing: At what time does it usually occur? How often?

☐ 2. Have you ever been hospitalized before? Any accidents or injuries? Allergies? Any similar episodes before?

☐ 3. Are your parents living? How's their health? How about your brothers and sisters? Do you have children? How's their health?

☐ 4. What is your occupation? Do you feel stressed at work? Do you use tobacco products? How about alcohol? Do you take any kind of recreational drugs? Who do you live with?

☐ 5. Now, I will be asking you some questions of a sensitive nature. I can assure you that anything you say will be kept confidential. I just need to ask these questions so I can have a clearer picture of your overall health. Are you sexually active? Are your partners men, women or both? How many partners have you had during the past year? Do you use condoms?

Thanks for answering these questions. Now I will be examining some parts of your body but let me wash my hands first. *(Wash hands.)* Let me put this drape on so you'll feel more comfortable. *(Drape patient.)*

☐ 6. I will be inspecting your belly.
☐ 7. Now I will be listening to your belly.
☐ 8. Can you show me with one finger exactly where the pain is?
☐ 9. I will be pressing on your belly. *(Watch for inspiratory arrest~Murphy's sign.)*
☐ 10. I will be pressing on other areas of your belly and you let me know if it hurts or not.
☐ 11. I will be tapping on your belly.
☐ 12. Does it hurt anywhere in your belly when I press this? *(Rovsing's sign)*
☐ 13. I will be bending and rotating your thigh and let me know if you feel any pain. *(Obturator sign)*
☐ 26. Can you lie on your left side? I will be stretching your thigh and let me know if you feel any pain. *(Psoas sign)*

Now let me summarize what you've told me. You said you have abdominal pain located in this area. My initial impression of your condition is acute cholecystitis — an inflammation of a small organ below the liver. But I am also considering other possibilities like hepatitis, peptic ulcer disease, etc. So I am ordering an ultrasound and some blood tests to make sure that we're on the right track. Do you have any questions?

Challenging Questions:

Is this related to pregnancy?
Is this related to the birth control pills I'm taking?
Is this related to menopause?
Is this the same illness I had a year ago?
What is acute cholecystitis?
What is a HIDA scan?
I have read in the Internet that taking *black cohosh* will help. Can I take this?
Why are you considering hepatitis when I don't look yellow?

Abdominal Pain (Acute Cholecystitis)

History:

cc:	abdominal pain
HPI:	– 42 y/o female complaining of RUQ pain that started 4 hrs. ago – crampy with radiation to right arm and shoulder – worsened by movement; not relieved by anything – pain progressively increasing from 5/10 to 9/10 on the pain scale – slight fever noted, no meds taken – (+) non-productive cough for 2 days
PMH:	– hospitalized a year ago for similar pain; was given medication that afforded relief; no h/o surgery; has Diabetes mellitus since age 30
FH:	brother has DM, other family members in good health
SocH:	– lives with husband and works as housekeeper; – smokes 1 ppd X 20 yrs; etoh (–), recreational drugs (–) – diet consists mainly of junk food
OB/GYN:	G2P2, all normal deliveries, LMP was 7 days ago No recent change in menses noted

Physical Examination:

Gen:	A&O, in pain
VS:	WNL except T 99.9° F
Skin:	no jaundice noted
Lungs:	clear BS, no rales, no rhonchi, N vocal and tactile fremitus
Abd:	– slightly protruberant, no cicatrix – NBS X 4 quadrants with N variation of tympany and dullness – (+) Murphy's sign ; (+) tenderness on RUQ on light and deep palpation; – no rebound tenderness; no hepatomegaly

Differential Diagnosis:

1. Acute cholecystitis
2. Hepatitis
3. Peptic Ulcer Disease
4. Acute Pancreatitis
5. Pneumonia

Diagnostic Work-ups:

1. Abdominal Ultrasound/HIDA scan
2. AST/ALT/AlkPhos/Total Bili
3. Amylase/Lipase
4. FOBT
5. Chest X-ray

CASE NO. 4

Mr. Peter Robinson is a 20-year-old male who complains of knee pain.

Vital Signs:

T 98.6° F
P 70
R 14
BP 125/85

EXPECTED TASKS

1. Gather the necessary clinical information.
2. Perform a focused and pertinent physical examination.
3. Discuss your diagnostic impressions and differential diagnosis with the patient.
4. Discuss work-ups to be ordered.
5. Complete the patient note after seeing the patient.

Knee Pain (Osteoarthritis)

(Knocks)

Hi, I'm Dr. ________ and I'm here to examine you today. Do you prefer to be called Mr. Robinson or Peter?

☐ 1. So, what brings you in today?
(Mnemonic: LMNOPQRST)
Location: Can you point with one finger exactly where the pain is?
Medications: Are you taking any medication right now?
Nausea and vomiting, weakness? Other symptoms?
Onset: When did this start?
Precipitating Factor: What makes it worse?
Quality: How would you describe the pain?
Radiation/**R**elieving Factors: Does it go anywhere? What makes it go away?
Severity: On a scale of 1–10, where 10 is the most painful, at what level would you rank your pain?
Timing: At what time does it usually occur? How often? How long does it last?

☐ 2. Have you had any fever recently? *(R/O septic arthritis.)*

☐ 3. Any history of trauma to this area?

☐ 4. Have you ever been hospitalized before? Any accidents or injuries? Allergies? Any similar episodes before?

☐ 5. Are your parents living? How's their health? How about your brothers and sisters? Do you have children? How's their health?

☐ 6. What is your occupation? Do you feel stressed at work? Do you use tobacco products? How about alcohol? Do you take any kind of recreational drugs? Who do you live with?

- ☐ 7. Now, I will be asking you some questions of a sensitive nature. I can assure you that anything you say will be kept confidential. I just need to ask these questions so I can have a clearer picture of your overall health. Is that okay with you? Are you sexually active? Are your partners men, women or both? How many partners have you had during the past year? Do you use condoms?

Thanks for answering these questions. Now I will be examining some parts of your body but let me wash my hands first. *(Wash hands.)* Let me put this drape on so you'll feel more comfortable. *(Drape patient.)*

- ☐ 8. I will be moving your lower leg and tell me to stop when it hurts. *(Range of motion.)*
- ☐ 9. Now I will be testing your knee. *(Anterior Drawer test and check for tenderness.)*
- ☐ 10. Now raise your thigh/leg/feet against my strength. Now, let's do it downward.
- ☐ 11. Let's check your reflexes now. *(Do biceps, triceps, knee and Achilles.)*
- ☐ 12. I will be bending your ankle. *(Homan's sign.)*
- ☐ 13. Now, I will be testing the other side. *(Always check the opposite, non-involved side.)*

Now let me summarize what you've told me. You said this pain started seven days go. Considering the history you told me and your physical examination, my initial impression of your condition is osteoarthritis — an inflammation or swelling of the knee joint due to wear and tear. But I am also considering other possibilities like rheumatoid arthritis, septic arthritis, torn ligament and SLE. So I am ordering some blood tests and imaging studies to make sure that we're on the right track. Do you have any questions?

Challenging Questions:

What is rheumatoid arthritis?
What herbal medicine can I take?
What is septic arthritis?
What is the life expectancy of people with lupus?
Is it possible that my girlfriend gave this to me?
What food should I stop eating?
What is SLE?

Knee Pain/Osteoarthritis

History:

cc:	knee pain
HPI:	20 y/o AAM, college basketball player c/o knee pain that started 4 days ago after a gym practice. Described as continuous, knife-like, exacerbated by walking or standing and relieved by non-usage. No medications taken aside from Ibuprofen q 6 hrs since yesterday which afforded temporary relief. Severity is 6/10 in the pain scale.
PMH:	no h/o of allergies, hospitalizations or accidents
FH:	unremarkable
SocH:	cig (–), etoh (–), illicit drugs (–)
SexH:	sexually active with girlfriend only, no h/o STD

Physical Examination:

Gen:	A&O X3, in pain
VS:	WNL
Skin:	normal color and turgor with no rashes noted
Musculoskeletal:	(+) tenderness of the R patellar area (–) Anterior Drawer Test Right Lower Extremity: Limited ROM, motor strength: 5/5 Sensory: intact, DTRs:++ Left Lower Extremity: Normal ROM, motor strength: 5/5 Sensory: intact, DTRs:++

Differential Diagnosis:

1. Osteoarthritis
2. Rheumatoid Arthritis
3. Septic Arthritis
4. Torn Ligament
5. SLE

Diagnostic Work-ups:

1. RF
2. ANA/anti-Smith/anti-dsDNA
3. CBC/ ESR
4. Synovial Fluid Analysis and C&S
5. X-ray of the knee joint

CASE NO. 5

Mr. Michael Donaldson is a 75-year-old white male who is complaining of shortness of breath.

Vital Signs:

T 98.0° F
P 101
R 25
BP 130/75

EXPECTED TASKS

1. Gather the necessary clinical information.
2. Perform a focused and pertinent physical examination.
3. Discuss your diagnostic impressions and differential diagnosis with the patient.
4. Discuss work-ups to be ordered.
5. Complete the patient note after seeing the patient.

Shortness of Breath

(Knocks)

Hi, I'm Dr. __________ and I'm here to examine you today. Do you prefer to be called Mr. Donaldson or Michael?

☐ 1. So, what brings you in today?
Do you have any problem breathing?
Any cough? Does it produce any gunk? What color? How often does this happen?
Can you walk without resting?
How many flights of stairs can you climb without stopping?
Do you have trouble breathing when lying on your back?
How many pillows do you use when you sleep?
Do you hear a wheezing sound when you breathe?
Do you feel any pain when you breathe?
When does it usually happen? How long does it last?
Any recent weight loss? Night sweats? Afternoon fever?

☐ 2. Have you ever been hospitalized before? Any accidents or injuries? Allergies? Any similar episodes of headache before?

☐ 3. Are your parents living? How's their health? How about your brothers and sisters? Do you have children? How's their health? Any history of asthma?

☐ 4. What is your occupation? Do you feel stressed at work? Do you use tobacco products? For how long? How about alcohol? Do you take any kind of recreational drugs? Who do you live with?

☐ 5. Now, I will be asking you some questions of a sensitive nature. I can assure you that anything you say will be kept confidential. I just need to ask these questions so I can have a clearer picture of your overall health. Is that okay with you? Are you sexually active? Are your partners men, women or both? How many partners have you had during the past year? Do you use condoms?

Thanks for answering these questions. Now I will be examining some parts of your body but let me wash my hands first. *(Wash hands.)* Let me put this drape on so you'll feel more comfortable. *(Drape patient.)*

☐ 6. I will be examining your chest.
☐ 7. Now, can you say "99" while I listen to your chest? Do that once again while I move my hands on various areas of your chest and back. *(Fremitus)*
☐ 8. I will be tapping on your chest.
☐ 9. I will be listening to your lungs. Breathe in and breathe out.
☐ 10. I would like to listen to your heart and feel your heartbeat.
☐ 11. I will now gently tap your sides. *(CVA tenderness)*
☐ 12. Now let's do the same to your back. *(Do inspection, fremitus, dullness and auscultation again on the posterior chest.)*
☐ 13. Can you inhale and hold it at the end while I tap your chest? Now breathe out and hold it at the end while I tap your chest. *(Diaphragmatic excursion)*

Now let me summarize what you've told me. You said you have this shortness of breath usually occurring _______. My initial impression of your condition is asthma. But I am also considering other possibilities like pneumonia, acute MI, COPD, and tension pneumothorax. We also want to be sure that we are not dealing with other problems, that's why I am ordering some procedures and tests. Do you have any questions?

Challenging Questions:

What is COPD?
What medication are you going to prescribe?
Don't you think I have a lung tumor?
Am I having a heart attack?
I don't smoke. Why would I have pneumonia?

Shortness of Breath (Asthma)

History:

cc:	shortness of breath
HPI:	75 y/o WM c/o shortness of breath (+) unproductive cough, (+) chest tightness, (+) recent URTI (–) colds, (–) fever, (–) rash symptoms were exacerbated by working in the garden no meds taken.
PMH:	same episode of shortness of breath several mos. ago that subsided after doctor gave some meds; previous h/o asthma; no accidents, no injuries
FamH:	father has asthma and smokes, CF (–), no heart disease
SocH:	lives with his wife, etoh (–), cig (–), illicit drugs (–)

Physical Examination:

Gen:	A&O
VS:	T: 98.0° F BP: 130/75 RR: 25 cpm HR: 101 bpm
CV:	NRRR, PMI not displaced, midclavicular line; no murmurs, gallops, rubs or clicks
Lungs:	symmetrical; wheezing (+) B/L, no rales, no dullness, normal vocal and tactile fremitus
Musculoskeletal:	No point tenderness on the anterior and posterior chest areas

Differential Diagnosis:

1. Asthma
2. COPD
3. Pneumonia
4. Acute MI
5. Tension Pneumothorax

Diagnostic Work-ups:

1. Pulse oximetry
2. EKG
3. CXR
4. Troponin/Myoglobin/CK-MB
5. PFT

CASE NO. 6

Ms. Jane Keaton is a 36-year-old female who came in complaining of fatigue.

Vital Signs:

T 98° F

P 70

R 14

BP 125/85

EXPECTED TASKS

1. Gather the necessary clinical information.
2. Perform a focused and pertinent physical examination.
3. Discuss your diagnostic impressions and differential diagnosis with the patient.
4. Discuss work-ups to be ordered.
5. Complete the patient note after seeing the patient.

Fatigue

(Knocks)

Hi, I'm Dr. _________ and I'm here to examine you today. Do you prefer to be called Ms. Keaton or Jane?

- ☐ 1. So, what brings you in today?
- ☐ 2. Onset: When did it start?
- ☐ 3. Do you have any trouble chewing or swallowing?
- ☐ 4. Do you have trouble adjusting to a temperature in a room? Do you prefer it warm or cold?
- ☐ 5. How's your appetite?
- ☐ 6. Have you noticed any weight changes lately?
- ☐ 7. Do you feel like you are thirsty all the time?
- ☐ 8. Do you feel like you want to pee all the time?
- ☐ 9. Have you noticed any changes in your hair recently?
- ☐ 10. Have you noticed any changes in the size of your shoes or hat?
- ☐ 11. How would you describe your mood?
- ☐ 12. When was the last time you had a blood count? What was the result?
- ☐ 13. Have you ever been hospitalized before? Any accidents or injuries? Allergies?
- ☐ 14. Are your parents living? How's their health? How about your brothers and sisters? Do you have children? How's their health?
- ☐ 15. What is your occupation? Do you feel stressed at work? Do you use tobacco products? For how long? How about alcohol? Do you take any kind of recreational drugs? Who do you live with?

- [ ] 16. I usually ask questions about sexual habits as part of my routine evaluation. Are you sexually active? Do you use any contraception? Have you ever had unprotected sex? Do you have sexual partners of the same sex, opposite sex or both? How many partners have you had during the past 12 months?

We've gone over a lot of information. Now I will be doing a physical examination but let me wash my hands first. *(Wash hands.)* Would you be more comfortable if I put this drape on your legs? *(Drape patient if she says yes.)*

- [ ] 17. I will be checking your eyes. *(pallor for anemia)*
- [ ] 18. I will be shining this light on your eyes. Just look straight while I do this. *(Funduscopic to R/O DM changes.)*
- [ ] 19. I will be examining your thyroid. *(Palpate thyroid)*
- [ ] 20. Can you put your chin down and slightly to the right? I will be pressing on this side *(displace larynx to the right side)* and I will ask you to swallow and I will try to feel your thyroid. OK, now swallow. Good. Now let's do it on the other side.
- [ ] 21. I will be listening to your neck. *(Carotid bruits)*
- [ ] 22. I would like to listen to your heart and lungs.

Now let me summarize what we have talked about. You came because of fatigue which was accompanied by weight gain of 15 pounds. Based on the history and the physical examination my initial impression of your condition is hypothyroidism. But I am also considering other possibilities like Diabetes mellitus, depression, anemia, and chronic fatigue syndrome. I will be ordering some test to make sure that we look at the different possibilities so we can make better decisions on how we will deal with your condition. Do you have any questions before I go?

Challenging Questions:

I don't have a sweet tooth. How can I have diabetes?
What do you think is wrong with my thyroid?
If it's a thyroid problem, why do I feel sad all the time?
Is this related to my previous ulcer problem?
Can I use water pills to shed some pounds?

Fatigue

History:

cc:	fatigue
HPI:	– 36 y/o WF c/o fatigue – started 7 days ago, usually occurring at the end of the day – weight gain of 15 lbs since 6 mos ago – normal appetite – bothered by cold weather – feels sad all the time – sleeps about 9 hrs/day – constipation 2x/week
PMH:	PUD diagnosed 4 years ago; cured as claimed
FamH:	father has diabetes; mother has hypertension
SocH:	works as a nurse assistant; job considered not stressful cig (–), etoh (–), drugs of abuse (–) sexually active with husband only

Physical examination:

Gen:	well-groomed, not in distress
VS:	WNL
HEENT:	tongue not enlarged
Neck:	thyroid not enlarged; no nodules; no tenderness no carotid bruits
Heart:	no murmurs, PMI not displaced, no JVD, no pedal edema, no cyanosis
Lungs:	unremarkable

Differential Diagnosis:

1. Hypothyroidism
2. Major Depression
3. Anemia
4. Chronic Fatigue Syndrome
5. Diabetes mellitus

Diagnostic Work-ups:

1. TSH/FT4/T3
2. CBC
3. Radioiodine scan
4. FBS
5. ECG

CASE NO. 7

Dr. Chris Gray is a 70-year-old retired male physician who complains of increased incidence of falling.

Vital Signs:

T 98° F
P 70
R 14
BP 125/85

EXPECTED TASKS

1. Gather the necessary clinical information.
2. Perform a focused and pertinent physical examination.
3. Discuss your diagnostic impressions and differential diagnosis with the patient.
4. Discuss work-ups to be ordered.
5. Complete the patient note after seeing the patient.

Parkinson's Disease

(Knocks)

Hi, Dr. Gray. I'm Dr. ________ and I'm here to examine you today.

- ☐ 1. So, what brings you in today?
- ☐ 2. Have you had any episodes of falling or tripping? Since when? How often?
- ☐ 3. Did you feel dizzy or did you feel a spinning sensation when you fell?
- ☐ 4. Did you pass out?
- ☐ 5. When did your tremors start? Any family member with the same kind of tremors?
- ☐ 6. Do you have any trouble getting dressed? How about eating, walking around or going to the bathroom?
- ☐ 7. Who does your shopping? How do you keep up with the daily household chores? Are all your bills up to date?
- ☐ 8. Have you had any illnesses or injuries in the past? Any allergies? Have you ever seen a psychiatrist? Did he prescribe any medication? *(R/O Drug-Induced Parkinsonism.)*
- ☐ 9. Are your family members in good health?
- ☐ 10. Do you use any tobacco products? Alcohol? How about recreational drugs?
- ☐ 11. How would you describe your mood? What do you do for recreation? Do you still like to do them now? Do you sleep well? Do you have trouble concentrating? Have you ever felt that you want to hurt yourself or somebody else? *(R/O Depression.)*
- ☐ 12. Any weight changes? What bothers you more, a hot or cold temperature? Any changes in your bowel movements? *(R/O Hypothyroidism.)*

☐ 13. Now I will be asking you some questions and will ask you to do some things that may challenge your thinking. This is important in making an assessment of your total health.

Where are you now?
What is today's date?
Who am I?
Who was the president before Ronald Reagan?
What did you have for breakfast this morning?
8 plus 7? 25 minus 3?
What do you understand when I say "time is money"?
Have you been seeing things other people don't see?

Ask about sexual history.

☐ 14. Now, I will be asking you some questions of a sensitive nature. I can assure you that anything you say will be kept confidential. I just need to ask these questions so I can have a clearer picture of your overall health. Is that okay with you? Are you sexually active? Are your partners ment, women or both? How many partners have you had during the past year? Do you use condoms?

Now I will be doing a physical exam but let me wash my hands first. *(Wash hands.)*

☐ 15. I will be holding your wrist. Now, can you bend your elbow? Now, try to straighten it. *(Cogwheeling)*

☐ 16. Can you get up from your chair and walk across the room and back? *(Get up and Go)*

☐ 17. Can you pick this object from my hand? *(Tremors decrease during activity.)*

☐ 18. Now I will try to feel your thyroid and let me now if you feel any pain when I do it, OK?

Thanks for answering all my questions. Now let me summarize. You told me that you have been falling… and that… You also said that you've had these tremors that… After doing this interview and a physical exam, I think we are dealing with Parkinson's Disease. But I am also considering other possibilities like depression, hypothyroidism, electrolyte imbalance, and brain tumor. I will be ordering a blood test to make sure that it is not your thyroid that's giving you this problem. Do you have any questions?

Challenging Questions:

What made you think this is a brain tumor?
What is essential tremor?
What test will you order for Parkinson's Disease?
If this is depression, can I take St. John's wort?
What causes Parkinson's Disease?

Parkinson's Disease

History

cc:	frequent falls
HPI:	62 y/o male c/o falling frequently since 6 mos. ago
	(–) prodrome, (–) unconsciousness, (–) vertigo
	ADLs impaired. IADLs impaired
	(+) lack of energy and reduced concentration, (+) tremors at rest
	(–) suicidal or homicidal ideation
	(–) intolerance to cold
PMH:	no h/o medical use including "mood medications"
FH:	no family h/o tremors
SocH:	cig (–), etoh (–), drugs of abuse (–)
SexH:	refuses to answer

Physical Examination:

Gen:	A&O X3, mask-like fascies
VS:	WNL
Neck:	thyroid has no tenderness, no nodules, no enlargement, no mass
Neuro:	(+) cogwheel rigidity, (+) get up and go test, (+) bradykinesia
	slow speech, (+) shuffling gait
	CN III-XII intact
	motor strength: 5/5 X4 extremities
	sensation: intact
	DTRs: ++ X4 extremities
MMSE:	unremarkable

Differential Diagnosis:

1. Parkinson's Disease
2. Major Depression
3. Hypothyroidism
4. Electrolyte imbalance
5. Brain Tumor

Diagnostic Work-ups:

1. Cranial CT scan
2. Lytes
3. TSH/FT4/T3
4. Magnesium/Phosphate/Calcium
5. FBS

CASE NO. 8

Mr. Jude Northfield is a 32-year-old male who came in complaining of diarrhea.

Vital Signs:

T 98.6° F
P 100
R 20
BP 120/85

EXPECTED TASKS

1. Gather the necessary clinical information.
2. Perform a focused and pertinent physical examination.
3. Discuss your diagnostic impressions and differential diagnosis with the patient.
4. Discuss work-ups to be ordered.
5. Complete the patient note after seeing the patient.

Diarrhea (Adult)

(Knocks)

Hi, I'm Dr. ________ and I'm here to ask you a few questions and do a physical exam. Do you prefer to be called Mr. Northfield or Jude?

☐ 1. So, what brings you in today?

(Mnemonic: Start ABCDEFG UVW)

Start: When did it start?

Aggravating/**A**lleviating/**A**ssociated symptoms: What makes it worse? What relieves it? Any fever, vomiting, tenesmus?

Blood: Is it bloody? *(Shigella, Salmonella,Campylobacter, IBD)*

Color/**C**onsistency: What's the color of your stool? Is it hard, soft or watery?

Duration/**D**iet: How long has it been going on? *(acute<3 weeks: viral, bacterial, drugs)* What did you eat before you start having diarrhea? *(Staph, B. cereus, C. perfringens)*

Episodes in the past: Any similar episodes in the past?

Frequency: How many times a day do you move your bowels?

Group Exposure: Anybody at home or at work with a similar problem?

Travel: Any history of travel, camping, swimming or hiking?

Use of Antibiotics/**L**axatives:

Have you taken any antibiotics recently? *(Pseudomembranous colitis)*

How about laxatives? *(Laxative abuse)*

Venereal Disease: Any history of STD? *(AIDS)*

Weight Loss: Have you lost any weight? Do you sweat a lot? Does a hot or cold temperature bother you? *(Hyperthyroidism)*

- ☐ 2. Have you had any illnesses in the past? Any allergies?
- ☐ 3. Any family member with the same problem you're having? Any history of bowel problems in the family? How about diabetes?
- ☐ 4. What is your occupation? Do you get stressed at work? Do you use any tobacco products? How about alcohol? How about recreational drugs?
- ☐ 5. I will be asking you some questions of a sensitive nature but is important in determining your total health. And everything will be kept confidential. Is that okay with you? Are you sexually active? Do you have sex with the same sex, opposite sex or both?

Now, I will be doing a physical examination but let me wash my hands first. *(Wash hands.)* This drape may help to make you a little more comfortable. *(Drape patient.)*

- ☐ 6. I will be feeling your heartbeat then I will listen to your heart with my stethoscope.
- ☐ 7. I will be listening to your belly and then I will be tapping it, OK?
- ☐ 8. Now, I will be pressing on your belly and let me know if it hurts, OK?
- ☐ 9. I will be tapping on your chest and your belly. *(liver span)*

Now, let me summarize what you have told me. You said that your diarrhea started ______. My inital impression of your condition is bacterial or viral gastroenteritis but I am also considering giardiasis-a different kind of bug that may also cause diarrhea. That is why I am ordering a stool exam to find out what is causing your diarrhea. I am also considering other possibilities like Inflammatory Bowel Disease, hyperthyroidism and cancer of the colon or rectum. That is why, in addition to stool exams I am also ordering a blood test, a rectal exam and a barium enema — a special kind of x-ray for the belly. Do you have any question?

Challenging Questions:

How did I get this?
Will taking Pepto-Bismol help?
Cancer? How bad is it?
How can a thyroid problem cause diarrhea?
What precautions should I take so my girlfriend won't get this, too?
Can I drink tea?
What should I eat?

Diarrhea

History

cc:	diarrhea
HPI:	– 32 y/o male college student c/o non-bloody diarrhea X 5 days
	– no h/o recent travel or eating in a big group
	– no h/o diarrhea in close contacts
	– colicky abdominal pain without radiation
	– not relieved by Loperamide
	– no fever noted
PMH:	– never been hospitalized
FH:	immediate family members apparently in good health
SocH:	– lives alone in an apartment
	– cig (–), etoh only during special occasions, recreational drugs (–)
	– diet consists mainly of junk food
SexH:	sex with girlfriend only

Physical Exam:

General:	A&O X3
VS:	T: 98.6° F BP: 120/85 RR: 20 PR: 100
HEENT:	eyes not sunken, mouth moist
GI:	increased bowel sounds X4 quadrants, no tenderness, no guarding, no rigidity, no hepatomegaly
Skin:	normal color and turgor

Differential Diagnosis

1. Bacterial or Viral Gastroenteritis
2. Giardiasis
3. Inflammatory Bowel Disease
4. Hyperthyroidism
5. Carcinoma of the colon or rectum.

Diagnostic Work-ups:

1. Stool analysis/culture/WBC/O&P
2. TSH
3. Rectal exam
4. CEA/barium enema
5. Biopsy of colon

CASE NO. 9

Mrs. Lakeisha Johnson is a 42-year-old female who was admitted with loss of consciousness.

Vital Signs:

T 98° F
P 87
R 18
BP 118/75

EXPECTED TASKS

1. Gather the necessary clinical information.
2. Perform a focused and pertinent physical examination.
3. Discuss your diagnostic impressions and differential diagnosis with the patient.
4. Discuss work-ups to be ordered.
5. Complete the patient note after seeing the patient.

Syncope/Seizure

(Knocks)

Hi, I'm Dr. __________ and I'm here to examine you today. *(Shakes patient's hand.)* By the way, do you prefer to be called Lakeisha or Mrs. Johnson?

- ☐ 1. So, what brings you in today?
  (Mnemonics: Start Before and After Rash PEF)
- ☐ 2. **Start:** When did this start?
- ☐ 3. **Before:** What were you doing before it happened?
- ☐ 4. **After:** Have you noticed anything unusual after it happened?
- ☐ 5. **Rash:** Did you notice any rash?
- ☐ 6. **Precipitating:** What do you think makes you start getting these attacks?
- ☐ 7. **Prodrome:** Do you feel anything unusual right before it happens?
- ☐ 8. **Pass out:** Did you lose consciousness?
- ☐ 9. **Prior episodes:** Has this ever happened before?
- ☐ 10. **Exposure:** Have you had recent contact with anyone who is ill?
- ☐ 11. **Electrolyte:** Any vomiting? Diarrhea? Are you taking water pills?
- ☐ 12. **Focal:** Did the attack involve just a part of your body or the entire body?
- ☐ 13. **Fever:** Do you have fever?
- ☐ 14. **Fluids:** Did you uncontrollably pee/poop/drool when this happened?

- ☐ 15. Have you had any accidents or injuries in the past? Any illnesses in the past? How about allergies? Any heart problems?
- ☐ 16. How's your parents' health? How about your brothers and sisters? Do you have kids? How's their health? Any family member with seizure disorder? Any family member with diabetes?

☐ 17. What type of job do you do? Do you drink alcoholic beverages? Do you smoke? Any use of recreational drugs?

☐ 18. I will be asking some questions of a sensitive nature that will help me better assess your total health. I can assure you that this will all be kept confidential. Is that okay with you? Are you sexually active? Do you use any contraception? Have you ever had unprotected sex? Do you have sexual partners of the same sex, opposite sex or both? How many partners have you had during the past 12 months?

We have discussed quite a lot. Now, I will be doing a physical examination but let me wash my hands first. *(Wash hands.)* Would you be more comfortable if I put this drape on your legs? *(Drape patient if she says yes.)*

☐ 19. Can you follow my finger without moving your head? *(Do EOM to test for CN III, IV, VI)*

☐ 20. I'll be touching several parts of your face and you touch them after I do it. *(Touch forehead, cheek and jaw.)*

☐ 21. Raise your eyebrows. Show your teeth. Smile. Puff your cheeks. Close your eyes and keep them closed while I try to open them. Close your mouth and keep it closed while I try to open it. Open your mouth and say "Ah!" Stick your tongue out. Point your tongue to the left. Point your tongue to the right.

☐ 22. Turn your head to the right against the strength of my hand. Let's do the same thing on the other side. Shrug your shoulder against my strength.

☐ 23. Raise your arm upward against my strength. Bring it downward against my strength. Now, we'll do the same for your hands and forearms.

☐ 24. Raise your thigh upward against my strength. Now bring it downward. We'll do the same for your legs and feet.

☐ 25. I will be touching parts of your arms and legs while your eyes are closed and I'd like you to point to the areas that I have touched. *(Sensory)*

☐ 26. Now I will be testing your reflexes. *(DTRs)*

☐ 27. Can you lie down for a minute? I'll be gently bending your neck forward. *(Note pain or resistance — Brudzinski)*

☐ 28. Now I will fold and straighten your knee. *(Kernig's)*

☐ 29. I will be stroking the sole of your foot. *(Babinski)*

☐ 30. Can you alternately touch your nose and my finger? *(Nose to finger test)*

☐ 31. Can you please stand up? Keep your feet close together and hands at your side. Close your eyes for a moment and don't open them until I say so. *(Romberg).*

☐ 32. I will be listening to your heart and lungs.

☐ 33. Now I will be asking you some question and will ask you to do some things that may challenge your thinking. This is important in making an assessment of your total health.

Where are you now?
What is today's date?
Who am I?
Who was the president before Ronald Reagan?
What did you have for breakfast this morning?
8 plus 7? 25 minus 3?
What do you understand when I say "time is money"?
Have you been seeing things other people don't see?

I think that's all for now. Let me summarize what we have talked about. You told me that your seizure attack started ______. So, right now my initial impression of your problem is what we call epilepsy — an abnormality in the electrical system of your body. But I am also looking at other problems in the brain which can be due to tumors or infections. There is also a possibility that we might be dealing with an electrolyte abnormality or imbalances in the chemical composition of your blood. Another possibility is a heart problem. I am looking at all these scenarios and I will be ordering some test to narrow down our search for what's giving you trouble. When the results are available I will see you again and we will discuss your condition and what your options are. Any question before I go?

Challenging Questions:

There's nobody in our family that has this.
Are you saying that I have brain cancer?
What do you mean by electrolyte abnormality?
Will drinking Gatorade help?
What causes epilepsy?

Syncope/Seizure

History:

cc:	loss of consciousness
HPI:	– 42 y/o AAF who lost consciousness accompanied by seizure yesterday
	– had a similar episode when she was 5 y/o
	– was on medication after that for a few years and meds discontinued by MD
	– was under stress at work
	– smelled something funny right before passing out; slight headache; no fever; no photophobia
PMH:	– hospitalized as a young girl for a single episode of seizure
FH:	immediate family members apparently in good health
SocH:	– lives with husband and 3 kids
	– cig (–), etoh (–), recreational drugs (–)
	– diet consists mainly of junk food
SexH:	sex with husband only; no h/o STD

Physical Exam:

General:	A&O X3, cooperative
VS:	WNL
HEENT:	scalp with no evidence of mass or trauma; fundi WNL
Heart:	no murmurs
Neuro:	CN II-XII intact, DTR normal, sensory intact, motor 4/4 X4 extremities; Kernig's (–), Brudzinski's (–); Babinski (–), Romberg (–)
MMSE:	normal findings

Differential Diagnosis:

1. Epilepsy
2. CNS tumor
3. Meningitis
4. Electrolyte imbalance
5. Heart Disease

Diagnostic Work-ups:

1. EEG
2. CT Scan
3. Lytes/Glucose/Ca^{++}
4. CSF Analysis
5. ECG

CASE NO. 10

Ms. Anne Marie Willard is a 24-year-old female who came in with menstrual cramps.

Vital Signs:

T 98.4° F
P 81
R 17
BP 138/78

EXPECTED TASKS

1. Gather the necessary clinical information.
2. Perform a focused and pertinent physical examination.
3. Discuss your diagnostic impressions and differential diagnosis with the patient.
4. Discuss work-ups to be ordered.
5. Complete the patient note after seeing the patient.

Menstrual Cramps

(Knocks)

Hi, I'm Dr. _____ and I'm here to examine you today. *(Shakes patient's hand.)* By the way, do you prefer to be called Anne Marie or Ms. Willard?

- ☐ 1. So, what brings you in today?
- ☐ 2. When did the pain start? What makes it worse? What makes it better? Has this happened before? How often?
- ☐ 3. Did you take any medication? Did you get relief from it?
- ☐ 4. When was the last day of your most recent menstrual period?
- ☐ 5. Have you noticed any changes in the amount and frequency of the flow?
- ☐ 6. At what age did you start having your periods?
- ☐ 7. Do you have a regular cycle? Every how many days?
- ☐ 8. Have you ever been pregnant? How many times?
- ☐ 9. How many children do you have? Any miscarriages? Any abortions?

I will be asking you some personal questions and I can assure you that your answers will be kept confidential. Your answers will give me a better understanding of what is bothering you.

- ☐ 10. Do you use any kind of contraception?
- ☐ 11. Have you ever had unprotected sex?
- ☐ 12. How many sexual partners have you had during the past 12 months? Are your partners of the same sex, opposite sex or both?
- ☐ 13. Do you have any history of sexually transmitted disease?
- ☐ 14. When was your most recent Pap smear? Do you know the results?

- ☐ 15. Do you feel any pain during sexual intercourse? Do you feel pain when you pee?
- ☐ 16. Do you think you are pregnant? Do you have any fever?
- ☐ 17. Have you been hospitalized before? Any history of accidents or injuries?
- ☐ 18. How's your parents' health? How about your brothers and sisters? Do you have kids? How's their health?
- ☐ 19. What type of job do you do? Do you drink alcoholic beverages? Do you smoke? Any use of recreational drugs?

Now, I will be doing a physical examination but let me wash my hands first. *(Wash hands.)* Would you be more comfortable if I put this drape on your legs? *(Drape patient if she says yes.)*

- ☐ 20. I will be inspecting your belly. Now, I will be listening to your belly.
- ☐ 21. Can you show me with one finger exactly where the pain is?
- ☐ 22. I will be pressing on your belly and you let me know if it hurts.
- ☐ 23. I will be tapping on your belly.
- ☐ 24. Does it hurt anywhere in your belly when I press this. *(Rovsing's sign)*
- ☐ 25. I will be bending and rotating your thigh and let me know if you feel any pain. *(Obturator sign)*
- ☐ 26. Can you lie on your left side? I will be stretching your thigh and let me know if you feel any pain. *(Psoas sign)*

I think that's all for now. Now, let me summarize what we have talked about. You told me that your menstrual cramps started ______. At this point I am considering the possibility of Premenstrual Dysphoric Disorder or PDD for short. This condition can be caused by hormonal changes and happens right before a woman gets her period. I am also considering other possibilities including pregnancy, UTI or bladder infection, appendicitis and pelvic inflammatory disease. I will be ordering some tests and once the results are back I will sit down with you and discuss these things further. Do you have any questions before I go?

Challenging Questions:

It's impossible that I am pregnant. We use condoms all the time.
Why are you ordering a pregnancy test?
A friend at school told me that this may be endometriosis. What's your take on this?
Is this the same as premenstrual syndrome?
Should I take a birth control pill to get rid of it?
Can I drink cranberry juice?

Menstrual cramps

History:

CC:	menstrual cramps
HPI:	– 24 y/o white female medical student c/o painful period – started 3 yrs ago with worsening progression – suprapubic incapacitating pain described as crampy and severe with occasional radiation to the back – Partially relieved by bed rest but not by Ibuprofen – LMP was 2 weeks ago; light flow (2–4 pads per day) – Pap smear a year ago was normal
PMH:	h/o fibroadenoma — surgically removed a year ago
FH:	father has hypertension
SocH:	lives in a dorm with a roommate; cig (–); etoh occasional, recreational drugs (–)
SexH:	Sexually active with 2 boyfriends using condoms all the time.
OB/Gyn:	G0P0

Physical Examination:

General:	A&O X3
VS:	WNL except BP 138/78
Abdomen:	slightly protruberant, N ABS X4 quadrants, N variation between dullness and tympany, no guarding, no organomegaly, Rovsing's (–), Psoas test (–), Obturator tests (–)

Differential Diagnosis:

1. PDD
2. Pregnancy
3. UTI
4. Appendicitis
5. Pelvic Inflammatory Disease (PID)

Diagnostic Work-ups:

1. Serum HCG
2. Urinalysis
3. Abdominal US
4. Pelvic exam
5. Vaginal culture

CASE NO. 11

Mr. Howard McDaniel is a 47-year-old male who came in for a routine annual physical examination.

Vital Signs:

T 99° F
P 80
R 16
BP 120/80

EXPECTED TASKS

1. Gather the necessary clinical information.
2. Perform a focused and pertinent physical examination.
3. Discuss your diagnostic impressions and differential diagnosis with the patient.
4. Discuss work-ups to be ordered.
5. Complete the patient note after seeing the patient.

Routine Physical Examination

(Knocks)

Hi, I'm Dr. ______ and I'm here to examine you today. *(Shakes patient's hand.)* By the way, do you prefer to be called Howard or Mr. McDaniel?

- [ ] 1. I understand that you are here for a physical examination. Do you have any problems in particular?
- [ ] 2. Are there any changes in your sleeping pattern? Any visual problems lately?
- [ ] 3. Is your hearing okay?
- [ ] 4. Any problems with your mouth or throat?
- [ ] 5. Do you feel any enlargement or any bumps in your neck?
- [ ] 6. Any weakness or numbness in your arms or legs?
- [ ] 7. Do you have any chest pain? Any breathing problems?
- [ ] 8. Any pain anywhere in your belly? Any changes in your bowel movements?
- [ ] 9. Any problems when you pee? Any abnormal bleeding or discharge?
- [ ] 10. What's it like at home?
- [ ] 11. Have you had any accidents or injuries in the past? Any illnesses in the past? How about allergies?
- [ ] 12. How are your parents' health? How about your brothers and sisters? Do you have kids? How's their health?
- [ ] 13. What type of job do you do? Any heavy lifting or bending? Is it stressful? Do you drink alcoholic beverages? Do you smoke? Any use of recreational drugs? What type of exercise do you do? How often do you do it?

☐ 14. I will be asking some questions of a sensitive nature that will help me better assess your total health. I can assure you that this will all be kept confidential. Is that okay with you? Are you sexually active? Do you use any contraception? Have you ever had unprotected sex? Do you have sexual partners of the same sex, opposite sex or both? How many partners have you had during the past 12 months?

Now, I will be doing a physical examination but let me wash my hands first. *(Wash hands.)* Would you be more comfortable if I put this drape on your legs? *(Drape patient if he says yes.)*

☐ 15. Can you open your mouth for me? Say "Ah"
☐ 16. I will be checking your neck. *(Check thyroid and for any lympadenopathy)*
☐ 17. I will be listening to your heart and lungs.
☐ 18. I will be touching and listening to your belly.
☐ 19. I will be doing some tests on your arms and legs.

I think that's all for now. Now, let me summarize what we have talked about. You basically are doing well but we will need to follow up and monitor more closely your ______ (depending on the physical examination findings). I will be ordering a blood test, a urine test and a chest x-ray. *(Order PSA, and FOBT if indicated.)* Do you have any questions before I go?

Challenging Questions:

What kind of blood test are you ordering?
Do you think I should continue with my Atkins Diet?
Why are you ordering all these tests?
How often should I exercise?

Routine Physical Examination

History:

cc:	routine PE
HPI:	– 47 y/o WM for routine exam – also complains of lack of appetite and 10-lb weight loss in the past 2 mos
PMH:	foot surgery during service in the military in his 20s
FH:	Father and mother both have Diabetes mellitus, type II.
SocH:	lives with a male partner, etoh (+), cig (+) 30 pack yrs, recreational drugs (–)
SexH:	uses condom every once in a while

Physical Examination:

General:	A&O X3, cooperative, not in acute distress
VS:	BP: 120/80 HR: 80 RR:16 T: 99° F
HEENT:	fundi WNL, N otoscopic findings BL; no nasal discharge or bleeding, tonsils not enlarged, no lymphadenopathy (cervical, postauricular, supraclavicular, occipital), no JVD, trachea midline, no carotid bruit, no thyroid enlargement, tenderness or nodules
Chest/Lungs:	symmetrical BL, N breath sounds BL, normal vocal & tactile fremitus, no dullness, clear breath sounds BL, no rales, no egophony, no wheezes
Heart:	N rate, regular rhythm, PMI not displaced; no murmurs, gallops, rubs or clicks; no S3/S4 noted
Abdomen:	NBS X4 quadrants, no organomegaly, no tenderness, no guarding, tympanitic to percussion,
Skin:	N color & turgor, no rashes, no tumors, no scars, no edema
Neuro:	5/5 motor strength X4, ++ DTR X 4, sensory intact X 4

Differential Diagnosis:

1. HIV
2. DM
3. Hypertension
4. BPH

Diagnostic Work-ups:

1. HIV ELISA
2. FBS/Urinalysis
3. Repeat BP
4. PSA/digital rectal exam
5. CXR

CASE NO. 12

Ms. Chrissy Allen is a 30-year-old female who has had rashes on her face and on her thighs.

Vital Signs:

T 98.3° F
P 72
R 15
BP 125/80

EXPECTED TASKS

1. Gather the necessary clinical information.
2. Perform a focused and pertinent physical examination.
3. Discuss your diagnostic impressions and differential diagnosis with the patient.
4. Discuss work-ups to be ordered.
5. Complete the patient note after seeing the patient.

Systemic Lupus Erythematosus

(Knocks)

Hi, I'm Dr. ______ and I'm here to examine you today. *(Shakes patient's hand.)* By the way, do you prefer to be called Chrissy or Ms. Allen?

- ☐ 1. What brings you in today?
- ☐ 2. Have you noticed any sores in your mouth lately?
- ☐ 3. Have you noticed any unusual rashes on your skin? How about rashes on your face?
- ☐ 4. Any achy joints?
- ☐ 5. Have you been having chest pains lately?
- ☐ 6. Have you noticed any unusual color in your urine?
- ☐ 7. Have you experienced any seizures?
- ☐ 8. Have you ever been told by a physician that you have problems in your blood?
- ☐ 9. Do you notice any changes in the color of your skin when exposed to the sun?
- ☐ 10. Have you had miscarriages?
- ☐ 11. Any fever? Night sweats? Weight loss?
- ☐ 12. Do you notice any color changes in your fingers when exposed to cold temperature?
- ☐ 13. Any changes in your hair?
- ☐ 14. Are you taking any kind of medication? Are you taking any medications for your heart?
- ☐ 15. Have you had any accidents or injuries in the past? Any illnesses in the past? How about allergies?

- ☐ 16. How are your parents' health? How about your brothers and sisters? Do you have kids? How's their health?
- ☐ 17. What type of job do you do? Any heavy lifting or bending? Is it stressful? Do you drink alcoholic beverages? Do you smoke? Any use of recreational drugs? What type of exercise do you do? How often do you do it?
- ☐ 18. I will be asking some questions of a sensitive nature that will help me better assess your total health. I can assure you that this will all be kept confidential. Is that okay with you? Are you sexually active? Do you use any contraception? Have you ever had unprotected sex? Do you have sexual partners of the same sex, opposite sex or both? How many partners have you had during the past 12 months?

We have already discussed quite a bit. Now, I will be doing a physical examination but let me wash my hands first. *(Wash hands.)* Would you be more comfortable if I put this drape on your legs? *(Drape patient if she says yes.)*

- ☐ 19. I would like to examine your skin. *(Look for rashes or tightness.)*
- ☐ 20. Can you open your mouth for me?
- ☐ 21. Now I will be examining your elbow, your wrist and your knee. *(Look for arthritis.)*
- ☐ 22. Now I would like to listen to your heart and your lungs.
- ☐ 23. Now let me check your kidneys. I will be tapping your sides and you tell me if they hurt or not. *(CVA tenderness.)*

I think that is all I need for now. Let me summarize what we have done and talked about. You told me that you have ______. So, right now, my initial impression of your condition is SLE also known as lupus — a kind of disorder of the immune system. I am also considering the possibility of other conditions like rheumatoid arthritis, septic arthritis, hyperthyroidism and discoid lupus. I will be ordering some lab tests so we'll have more information. Do you have any questions?

Challenging Questions:

What causes lupus?
I need to go to the restroom.
What is discoid lupus?
What kind of blood tests are you ordering?
What is the immune system?
What does arthritis have to do with my rashes?

Systemic Lupus Erythematosus

History:

cc:	rash on face and thigh
HPI:	30 y/o female c/o butterfly rash on the face and thigh since 2 mos. ago. (+) arthralgia of R knee joint; (+) palpitations; N blood count 2 yrs ago; (+) photosensitivity; (+) fever at 100 F q 2 days usually in the afternoon and evening; (+) Reynauds phenomenon; (+) hair loss; (+) weight loss of 10 lbs in the past 2 mos.; (+) insomnia. No voice changes, no constipation, no miscarriages No cough, no SOB, no seizure, no numbness, no weakness, no hoarseness
PMH:	no h/o SLE, not on any kind of medication
FH:	no family h/o collagen vascular disease
SocH:	cig (–), etoh (–), drugs of abuse (–)
SexH:	(+) h/o syphilis; 2 sexual partners for the past 12 mos
OB/GYN:	G1P1

Physical Examination:

Gen:	A&O, not in pain or distress
VS:	WNL
Skin:	(+) butterfly rash on cheeks, (+) discoid rash
HEENT:	(+) alopecia, no thyroid nodules, tenderness or enlargement
Heart:	no murmurs or clicks
Lungs:	clear to auscultation B/L
Knee joint:	reduced ROM B/L with slight tenderness neg for balloon and bulge tests

Differential Diagnosis:

1. SLE
2. RA
3. Septic Arthritis
4. Hyperthyroidism
5. Discoid Lupus

Diagnostic Work-ups:

1. ANA/anti-Smith/anti-dsDNA
2. X-ray of knee joint (AP & Lat)
3. CBC/ESR/Uric acid/RF
4. TSH/FT4/T3
5. Knee joint fluid analysis and C&S

CASE NO. 13

Mrs. Edna Bautista is a 58-year-old female who came in because of eye pain.

Vital Signs:

T 98.4° F
P 90
R 20
BP 100/70

EXPECTED TASKS

1. Gather the necessary clinical information.
2. Perform a focused and pertinent physical examination.
3. Discuss your diagnostic impressions and differential diagnosis with the patient.
4. Discuss work-ups to be ordered.
5. Complete the patient note after seeing the patient.

Eye Pain

(Knocks)

Hi, I'm Dr. ______ and I'm here to examine you today. *(Shakes patient's hand.)* Do you prefer to be called Edna or Mrs. Bautista?

- ☐ 1. What brings you in today?
  (Mnemonic: SHADE I TUVWX)
- ☐ 2. **S**udden or chronic: Did this occur suddenly or has it been occurring for a long time?
- ☐ 3. **H**alos/**H**eadaches: Do you see any halos around lights? Do you have headaches?
- ☐ 4. **A**nticholinergics: Have you been taking any kind of medication?
- ☐ 5. **D**ischarge/**D**rugs: Have you noticed any discharge from your eye? Are you taking any medication right now?
- ☐ 6. **E**pisodes in the past: Have you had this problem before?
- ☐ 7. **I**tching: Does it itch?
- ☐ 8. **T**rauma: Did you have any accident or injury that might have affected your eye?
- ☐ 9. **U**nilateral or Bilateral: Is this problem affecting only one eye or both eyes?
- ☐ 10. **V**isual Loss/Vomiting & Nausea: Any loss of vision? How about nausea and vomiting?
- ☐ 11. **W**atery Eyes: Do your eyes feel watery most of the time?
- ☐ 12. **X**erophthalmia: Do your eyes feel dry most of the time?

- ☐ 13. Tell me what illnesses you have had in the past. Any hospitalizations? Allergies?

- ☐ 14. Any family history of diabetes? Hypertension? Are your parents in good health? How about your brothers and sisters? And your children?
- ☐ 15. What type of job do you do? Any heavy lifting or bending? Is it stressful? Do you drink alcoholic beverages? Do you smoke? Any use of recreational drugs? What type of exercise do you do? How often do you do it?
- ☐ 16. I will be asking some questions of a sensitive nature that will help me better assess your total health. I can assure you that this will all be kept confidential. Is that okay with you? Are you sexually active? Do you use any contraception? Have you ever had unprotected sex? Do you have sexual partners of the same sex, opposite sex or both? How many partners have you had during the past 12 months?

We've reviewed a lot of information. Now, I will be doing a physical examination but let me wash my hands first. *(Wash hands.)* Would you be more comfortable if I put this drape on your legs? *(Drape patient if she says yes.)*

- ☐ 17. I will be shining a light into your eyes. Can you look at the tip of my finger? Now look at the wall behind me. Then look at the tip of my finger again. *(PERLA)*
- ☐ 18. Follow my finger with your eyes without moving your head. *(EOM)*
- ☐ 19. I will be using this instrument to look into your eyes. *(Funduscopic exam)*
- ☐ 20. I will be examining your stomach. *(Inspection, auscultation, palpation, percussion)*

My initial impression of your condition is glaucoma. But I am also entertaining the possibilities of other illnesses including bacterial conjunctivitis, allergic conjunctivitis, corneal injury and uveitis. I am ordering a few tests for your eye, a blood test and a swab test. Do you have any questions before I go?

Challenging Questions:

What causes glaucoma?
What is uveitis?
What eyedrops do you recommend?
Is this infectious?
Am I going blind?
What kind of tests are you ordering?
Why are my eyes red?

Eye Pain

History:

cc:	eye pain
HPI:	58 y/o Asian female c/o eye pain of 1 hr duration (+) blurry vision, (+) halos around lights, (+) nausea (–) vomiting, (+) abdominal pain, (–) fever, (–) rash no meds taken.
PMH:	same episode of shortness of breath a year ago that subsided spontaneously without meds. no allergies, no accidents, no injuries
FamH:	father has asthma and smokes, CF (–), no heart disease
SocH:	(–) cig, (–) etoh, (–) illicit drugs

Physical Examination:

Gen:	A&O, in acute pain and distress
VS:	T: 98.4° F BP: 100/70 RR: 20 cpm HR: 90 bpm
HEENT:	(+) conjunctival injection; moderately dilated pupils; pupils non reactive to light; no discharge
Abdomen:	NABS; no tenderness, no rigiditiy, no organomegaly

Differential Diagnosis:

1. Glaucoma
2. Bacterial Conjunctivitis
3. Allergic Conjunctivitis
4. Corneal injury
5. Uveitis

Diagnostic Work-ups:

1. Tonometry
2. Swab for C&S
3. Eosinophil Count
4. Slit Lamp
5. Schirmer's Test

CASE NO. 14

Ms. Susan Riley is a 43-year-old female who has had difficulty swallowing for the past 6 months.

Vital Signs:

T 98° F
P 68
R 15
BP 120/70

EXPECTED TASKS

1. Gather the necessary clinical information.
2. Perform a focused and pertinent physical examination.
3. Discuss your diagnostic impressions and differential diagnosis with the patient.
4. Discuss work-ups to be ordered.
5. Complete the patient note after seeing the patient.

Dysphagia

(Knocks)

Hi, I'm Dr. __________. How are you today? *(Shakes patient's hand.)* I'm here to examine you and ask you a few questions. By the way, do you prefer to be called Susan or Ms. Riley?

☐ 1. So, what brings you in today?
☐ 2. Onset: When did you start having this problem?
☐ 3. Dysphagia/Odynophagia: Do you have difficulty swallowing? Is there pain when you swallow?
☐ 4. Solid/Liquid: Do you have difficulty swallowing solids, liquids or both?
☐ 5. Weight Loss: Have you noticed any change in your weight recently?
☐ 6. Hoarseness: Have you noticed any changes in your voice recently?
☐ 7. Reflux: Do you feel like the food you are eating is backflushing to your throat or mouth?
☐ 8. Alcohol/Tobacco: Do you drink alcoholic beverages? Do you smoke?
☐ 9. Chest Pain: Do you have any chest pains?
☐ 10. Have you had any illnesses in the past? Any accidents or allergies?
☐ 11. I will be asking you about diseases in the family, OK? Are your parents still healthy? How about your brothers and sisters? How about your husband and children?
☐ 12. What kind of work do you do? Do you use any recreational drugs?

- ☐ 13. Now, I will be asking you some questions of a sensitive nature. I can assure you that anything you say will be kept confidential. I need to ask these questions so I can have a clearer picture of your overall health status. Are you sexually active? Are your partners men, women or both? How many partners have you had during the past year? Do you use condoms?

Thanks for answering all these questions. At this point, I will be doing a physical examination but let me wash my hands first. *(Wash hands.)* Would you be more comfortable if I put this drape on your legs? *(Drape patient if she answers yes.)*

- ☐ 14. Can you open your mouth so I can take a look? Say "Ahhhh."
- ☐ 15. Now let me examine your neck for bumps or swollen areas. *(Note cervical lymphadenopathy)*
- ☐ 16. Let me check your thyroid.
- ☐ 17. I would like to listen to your chest.

Now let me summarize what we have talked about. You came because of a difficulty in swallowing that started ______. Based on the history and the physical examination my initial impression of your condition is a narrowing of the food passages — a condition called achalasia. But I am also considering other possibilities and I will be ordering some tests to make sure that we consider all the possibilities. Do you have any questions?

Challenging Questions:

What is achalasia?
What causes it?
What is an esophagogram?
What are the chances that this is cancer?
What kind of tests are you ordering?
Will I be needing surgery?

Dysphagia

History:

cc:	dysphagia
HPI:	43 y/o female c/o difficulty of swallowing both liquids and solids for 6 mos (+) regurgitation (+) 8-lb weight loss, (+) cough (+) chest pain, (–) fever, (–) shortness of breath no meds taken.
PMH:	no allergies, no accidents, no injuries
FamH:	father has asthma and smokes, CF (–), no heart disease
SocH:	lives alone, cig (–), etoh (–), illicit drugs (–)

Physical Examination:

Gen:	A&O
VS:	WNL
HEENT:	tongue midline with N size, color & texture; no ulcers or tumors; no buccal or pharyngeal erythema; no bleeding gums, tonsils not enlarged, no whitish plaques
Neck:	no lymphadenopathy (cervical, postauricular, supraclavicular, occipital), no JVD, trachea midline, no carotid bruit, no thyroid enlargement, tenderness or nodules
CV:	NRRR, PMI not displaced; no murmurs, gallops, rubs or clicks
Lungs:	symmetrical; wheezing (–) B/L, no rales, no dullness, normal vocal and tactile fremitus
Musculoskeletal:	No point tenderness on the anterior and posterior chest areas

Differential Diagnosis:

1. Achalasia
2. Esophageal CA
3. Diffuse esophageal spasm
4. Scleroderma
5. Hyperthyroidism

Diagnostic Work-ups:

1. Esophagogram
2. Esophageal pH monitoring
3. Endoscopy & Biopsy
4. TSH/FT4/T3
5. Anti-Scl-70

CASE NO. 15

Mr. Ronald Salvador is a 55-year-old male who came in complaining of frequent urination.

Vital Signs:

T 98.6° F
P 86
R 18
BP 130/80

EXPECTED TASKS

1. Gather the necessary clinical information.
2. Perform a focused and pertinent physical examination.
3. Discuss your diagnostic impressions and differential diagnosis with the patient.
4. Discuss work-ups to be ordered.
5. Complete the patient note after seeing the patient.

Diabetes Mellitus

(Knocks)

Hi, I'm Dr. ______ . How are you today? *(Shakes patient's hand.)* I'm here to examine you and ask you a few questions. By the way, do you prefer to be called Ronald or Mr. Salvador?

(Mnemonic: Onset PPP DIABETIC)

- ☐ 1. **Onset:** When did it start?
- ☐ 2. **P**olyuria: Do you pee a lot?
- ☐ 3. **P**olyphagia with weight loss: How's your appetite? Any changes in your weight?
- ☐ 4. **P**olydipsia: Do you get thirsty a lot?
- ☐ 5. **D**izziness on standing: Do you get dizzy when you suddenly stand up?
- ☐ 6. **I**mpotence: Do you have problem achieving or maintaining an erection?
- ☐ 7. **A**lcohol use: Do you drink alcoholic beverages?
- ☐ 8. **B**lurred vision: Do you have any problems with your vision?
- ☐ 9. **T**ingling or numbness of feet: Do you feel any tingling or numbness in your feet?
- ☐ 10. **I**ncontinence: Do you have trouble controlling your bladder
- ☐ 11. **C**laudication: Do you feel any pain in your legs when you walk?
- ☐ 12. Have you had any accidents or injuries in the past? Any illnesses in the past? How about allergies?
- ☐ 13. How are your parents' health? How about your brothers and sisters? Do you have kids? How's their health?

- ☐ 14. What type of job do you do? Any heavy lifting or bending? Is it stressful? Do you drink alcoholic beverages? Do you smoke? Any use of recreational drugs? What type of exercise do you do? How often do you do it?
- ☐ 15. I will be asking some questions of a sensitive nature that will help me better assess your total health. I can assure you that this will all be kept confidential. Is that okay with you? Are you sexually active? Do you use any contraception? Have you ever had unprotected sex? Do you have sexual partners of the same sex, opposite sex or both? How many partners have you had during the past 12 months?

We have gone over a lot of information. Now, I will be doing a physical examination but let me wash my hands first. *(Wash hands.)* Would you be more comfortable if I put this drape on your legs? *(Drape patient if he says yes.)*

- ☐ 16. I will be shining this light on your eyes. Just look straight while I do this. *(funduscopic)*
- ☐ 17. I will be listening to your neck. *(Carotid bruits)*
- ☐ 18. I would like to listen to your heart and lungs.
- ☐ 19. I will be touching several parts of your legs and feet with the dull and the sharp ends of this instrument. Tell me if it feels dull or sharp. *(Sensory of lower extremities)*

Now let me summarize what we have talked about. You came in because of problems about vision, peeing and weakness that started ______. Based on the history and the physical examination my initial impression of your condition is Diabetes mellitus — an uncontrolled elevation of blood sugar. But I am also considering other possibilities including hypertension, thyroid dysfunction, glaucoma, cataract, and anemia. I will be ordering some test to make sure that we consider all the possible scenarios so we can make better decisions on how we will deal with your condition. Do you have any questions before I leave?

Challenging Questions:

What causes diabetes?
A friend who is diabetic pokes himself everyday to test his sugar. Will I be doing that, too?
What is insulin?
Why do you pee a lot when your blood sugar is high?
Why will I have diabetes when nobody in our family has it?
If I lose weight, will my diabetes go away?
What kind of blood tests are you ordering?
Should I tell my children to get tested, too?
Should I stop eating anything sweet?
If this is really diabetes, I'm afraid of becoming impotent.

Diabetes Mellitus

History:

cc:	polyuria
HPI:	55 y/o Hispanic male c/o frequent urination (+) polyuria; (+) polydipsia; (+) polyphagia (–) impotence; (–) blurry vision; (–) tingling or numbness; no incontinence; no claudication; no fever no meds taken.
PMH:	no allergies, no accidents, no injuries; no h/o hospitalization
FamH:	father has diabetes and mother has hypertension
SocH:	cig (–); etoh occasional; illicit drugs (–)
SexH:	sex with wife only without protection

Physical Examination:

Gen:	A&O
VS:	WNL except BP 130/80
HEENT:	unremarkable funduscopic exam
CV:	NRRR, PMI not displaced; no murmurs, gallops, rubs or clicks; no carotid bruits
Musculoskeletal:	sensory of lower extremities intact

Differential Diagnosis:

1. Diabetes mellitus
2. Hypertension
3. Hypothyroidism
4. Cataract/Glaucoma
5. Anemia

Diagnostic Work-ups:

1. FBS
2. Repeat BP
3. TSH
4. CBC
5. Tonometry

CASE NO. 16

Mr. Zach Thomas is a 68-year-old male who came in complaining of back pain.

Vital Signs:

T 98.4° F
P 71
R 15
BP 120/80

EXPECTED TASKS

1. Gather the necessary clinical information.
2. Perform a focused and pertinent physical examination.
3. Discuss your diagnostic impressions and differential diagnosis with the patient.
4. Discuss work-ups to be ordered.
5. Complete the patient note after seeing the patient.

Back Pain

(Knocks)

Hi, I'm Dr. ________ and I'm here to examine you today. *(Shakes patient's hand.)* By the way, do you prefer to be called Zach or Mr. Thomas?

☐ 1. So what brings you in today?
(Mnemonic: LMNOPQRST)
☐ 2. **L**ocation: Can you tell me exactly where the pain is?
☐ 3. **M**edications: Have you taken any medications for it?
☐ 4. **N** & V and other symptoms: Do you have leg cramps? *(Spinal stenosis)*
☐ 5. **O**nset: When did it start?
☐ 6. **P**recipitating factor: What makes it worse?
☐ 7. **Q**uality: How would you describe the pain?
☐ 8. **R**adiation/**R**elieving Factors: Does it go anywhere? What makes it better? *(Leaning forward relieves spinal stenosis.)*
☐ 9. **S**everity: On a scale of 1–10 where ten is the most painful, where would you rank this pain?
☐ 10. **T**iming: What particular time of the day does the pain occur?

☐ 11. Have you had any accidents or injuries in the past? Any illnesses in the past? How about allergies?
☐ 12. How are your parents' health? How about your brothers and sisters? Do you have kids? How's their health?
☐ 13. What type of job do you do? Any heavy lifting or bending? Is it stressful? Do you drink alcoholic beverages? Do you smoke? Any use of recreational drugs? What type of exercise do you do? How often do you do it?

☐ 14. I will be asking some questions of a sensitive nature that will help me better assess your total health. I can assure you that this will all be kept confidential. Is that okay with you? Are you sexually active? Do you use any contraception? Have you ever had unprotected sex? Do you have sexual partners of thc samc sex, opposite sex or both? How many partners have you had during the past 12 months?

We've reviewed a lot of information. Now, I will be doing a physical examination but let me wash my hands first. *(Wash hands.)* Would you be more comfortable if I put this drape on your legs? *(Drape patient if he says yes.)*

☐ 15. I would like you to lie down on your back. Let me help you. *(Assists patient.)* Let me pull this extension for your legs. I will be raising your right leg and try not to bend your knee. I want it straight when I raise it. Here we go. Did you feel pain in your back? Now I will be crossing your leg to the other side and raising it again. Any pain when I do that? Now, I'll be doing the same tests on your other leg. *(Straight Leg Raising & Crossed Straight Leg Raising Test to r/o Sciatic Nerve Irritation and Herniated Disk.)*

☐ 16. Now can you sit up and let your legs hang loose. Let me push this leg extension back in place. *(Push leg extension in.)* Here, let me help you. *(Assists patient in getting up.)* I will be pressing on your spine and back, let me know if you feel any pain. *(Point tenderness)*

☐ 17. I will be testing your muscle strength. Can you raise your thigh/leg/foot up/down against my hand? *(Motor)*

☐ 18. I will be touching parts of your thighs, legs and feet, let me know if you feel them. *(Sensory)*

☐ 19. Now I will be testing your reflexes. *(Patellar & Achilles Reflex.)* I will be scratching the sole of your foot. *(Babinski)*

☐ 20. Now can you stand up. I will be holding your hips and will ask you to do several motions and you tell me if you feel any pain. Bend forward. Bend backward, please. Bend to your right side. Bend to your left side, please. Twist your shoulders to the right. Twist your shoulders to the left. *(ROM)*

☐ 21. Now can you walk across the room? Can you walk on your heels? Can you walk on your toes? *(Gait)*

I think that's all we have to do for now. Now, let me summarize what we have talked about. You told me that your back pain started ______. My initial impression of your problem is acute lumbosacral sprain. But I am also considering sciatic nerve irritation, herniated disc, osteoarthritis and prostatic carcinoma. I will be ordering some blood tests, some procedures to take picture of your spine and a rectal exam. Do you have any questions before I go?

If patient is young, consider spinal stenosis (relieved by leaning forward) and ankylosing spondylitis (with arthritis and uveitis) instead of osteoarthritis and prostatic CA. Add HLA-B27 in the lab orders.

Challenging Questions:

What is lumbosacral sprain?
Is sprain the same as strain?
Is there something wrong with my sciatic nerve?
Is this sciatica?
What do you think is wrong with my spine?
Is there an arthritis of the spine?
What? Possibly cancer of the prostate?
How bad is it?
What do you think? Is this cancer or not?

Back Pain

History:

cc:	back pain
HPI:	– 68 y/o WM c/o back pain that started 1 day ago after picking up his groceries
	– worsened by bending and sitting, relieved by lying down
	– sharp and 7/10 on the pain scale
	– (+) difficulty when walking but no numbness on lower extremities;
	– no radiation noted
	– no bowel or urine incontinence
PMH:	– gallstones removed 5 years ago
	– lung CA (–), knee pain (–), wrist pain (–)
FH:	– father died of heart disease
	– brother has knee pain with fever at present
SocH:	– doesn't exercise, drinks beer 1–2 bottles/week
	– sedentary lifestyle, cig (–), drugs of abuse (–)

Physical Examination:

Gen:	alert but in acute pain
VS:	WNL
Musculoskeletal:	tenderness on lumbosacral area by light and deep palpation; (–) straight leg raising test; HIP ROM reduced; normal gait; (–) CVA tenderness;
	motor: 5/5 on all 4 extremities
	sensory: intact on all 4 extremities
	reflex: ++ on all 4 extremities

Differential Diagnosis:

1. Acute lumbosacral sprain
2. Sciatic nerve irritation
3. Herniated disk
4. Osteoarthritis
5. Prostate CA

Diagnostic Work-ups:

1. MRI (lumbosacral)
2. X-ray (lumbosacral)
3. Digital Rectal Exam
4. PSA
5. Urinalysis

CASE NO. 17

Mr. Danny Flores is a 44-year-old male who came in with a generalized rash.

Vital Signs:

T 98.7° F
P 102
R 18
BP 120/85

EXPECTED TASKS

1. Gather the necessary clinical information.
2. Perform a focused and pertinent physical examination.
3. Discuss your diagnostic impressions and differential diagnosis with the patient.
4. Discuss work-ups to be ordered.
5. Complete the patient note after seeing the patient.

Rash/Allergic Reaction

(Knocks)

Hi, I'm Dr. ________ and I'm here to examine you today. *(Shakes patient's hand.)* By the way, how do you prefer to be called Danny or Mr. Flores?

- ☐ 1. So, what brings you in today?
- ☐ 2. When did this start?
- ☐ 3. What had you eaten before the rashes appeared?
- ☐ 4. Are you taking any medication?
- ☐ 5. What type of job do you do?
- ☐ 6. Have you noticed a problem with your neck recently? Any stiffness in your neck?
- ☐ 7. Any painful joints?
- ☐ 8. Have you been outdoors lately? Have you gone hiking recently? Where?
- ☐ 9. Do you have fever? Fatigue? Headache?
- ☐ 10. Have you been bitten by an insect?
- ☐ 11. Have you noticed any part of your skin becoming itchy lately?
- ☐ 12. Do you have muscle pains? How about muscle weakness?
- ☐ 13. Do you sometimes feel as if you are hearing your heartbeat?
- ☐ 14. Do you have a sore throat? Any shortness of breath?
- ☐ 15. Have you had any accidents or injuries or illnesses in the past? How about allergies? Rheumatic fever? STD?
- ☐ 16. How are your parents' health? How about your brothers and sisters? Do you have kids? How's their health?

- ☐ 17. What type of job do you do? Is it stressful? Do you drink alcoholic beverages? Do you smoke? Any use of recreational drugs? What type of exercise do you do? How often do you do it?
- ☐ 18. I will be asking some questions of a sensitive nature that will help me better assess your total health. I can assure you that this will all be kept confidential. Is that okay with you? Are you sexually active? Do you use any contraception? Have you ever had unprotected sex? Do you have sexual partners of the same sex, opposite sex or both? How many partners have you had during the past 12 months?

We've discussed a lot of information. Now, I will be doing a physical examination but let me wash my hands first. *(Wash hands.)* Would you be more comfortable if I put this drape on your legs? *(Drape patient if he says yes.)*

- ☐ 19. I will be examining your skin.
- ☐ 20. I will be examining your elbows and knees.
- ☐ 21. I will be listening to your heart and lungs.
- ☐ 22. I will be examining your neck.

Now let me summarize what we have talked about. You came in because of these rashes that started ______. Based on the history and the physical examination, my initial impression of your condition is what we call angioedema — some kind of allergic reaction. But I am also considering other possibilities including drug reaction, insect bite, hepatitis B, and parasitic infection. I will be ordering some tests for more information. Do you have any questions before I leave?

Challenging Questions:

What is angioedema?
What causes it?
How can I have a parasite? I've never been out of the United States.
I never do drugs and I'm not on any medication.
Insect bites don't look like this!
Hepatitis B? Isn't that sexually transmitted?

Rash/Allergic Reaction

History:

cc:	rash
HPI:	44 y/o Hispanic male c/o rash
	started 45 mins. ago after eating shellfish
	(+) itching, (–) fever, (–) fatigue, (–) headache
	no h/o if insect bite; no meds taken
	(–) sore throat, (–) shortness of breath, (–) muscle pains
	(–) arthralgia, (–) h/o outdoor activities
PMH:	no hospitalizations, no injuries, no trauma
	(+) h/o childhood asthma
FamH:	father has heart problems; mother has hypertension
SocH:	works as a grocery store manager
	Cig (–), etoh (–), illicit drugs (–)
SexH:	unprotected sex with wife only

Physical Examination:

Gen:	A&O
VS:	WNL except T: 98.7° F and HR: 102 bpm
CV:	NRRR, PMI not displaced; no murmurs, gallops, rubs or clicks
Lungs:	symmetrical; wheezing (+) B/L, no rales, no dullness, normal vocal and tactile fremitus
Skin:	generalized erythema and wheals, (–) jaundice

Differential Diagnosis:

1. Angioedema
2. Drug reaction
3. Insect bite
4. Hepatitis B
5. Parasitic infection

Diagnostic Work-ups:

1. CBC with diff
2. HBsAg/ALT
3. Stool ova and parasite
4. Specific drug level
5. Skin biopsy

CASE NO. 18

Ms. Karen Paxton is a 22-year-old white female complaining of a sore throat.

Vital Signs:

T 100° F
P 100
R 20
BP 125/85

EXPECTED TASKS

1. Gather the necessary clinical information.
2. Perform a focused and pertinent physical examination.
3. Discuss your diagnostic impressions and differential diagnosis with the patient.
4. Discuss work-ups to be ordered.
5. Complete the patient note after seeing the patient.

Sore Throat

(Knocks)

Hi, I'm Dr. ________. How are you today? *(Shakes patient's hand.)* I'm here to examine you and ask you a few questions. By the way, do you prefer to be called Karen or Ms. Paxton?

- ☐ 1. So, what brings you in today? *(Mnemonic: Start ABCDEFG)*
- ☐ 2. **Start:** When did it start? *(If > 1 week consider rheumatic fever.)*
- ☐ 3. **A**bdominal pain/**A**chy joints: Do you feel any swelling or pain in your stomach? Any painful joints?
- ☐ 4. **B**owel movement change/**Bl**ood Transfusion: Have you noticed any changes in your bowel movements? Any history of blood transfusion? *(R/O hepatitis and AIDS.)*
- ☐ 5. **C**ough/**C**ervical Lymaphadenopathy: Do you have a cough? Have you noticed any tender bumps on your neck? Is it painful when you swallow?
- ☐ 6. **D**uration/**D**iscoloration of skin: How long has this been going on? Have you had any rashes?
- ☐ 7. **E**xudate: Have you noticed any pus or gunk in your spit or in your throat?
- ☐ 8. **F**ever: Have you had any fever?
- ☐ 9. **G**roup Exposure: Do you have anybody you live with or any co-worker with the same problem? How about sexual partners? *(R/O adenovirus or Infectious mono.)*
- ☐ 10. Have you had any illnesses in the past? Have you ever been told by a doctor that you have hepatitis? *(R/O hepatitis.)* Are your immunizations complete? *(R/O Diphtheria.)*

- ☐ 11. I will be asking you about diseases in the family, OK? Do your parents have any health problems? How about your brothers and sisters? How about your kids?
- ☐ 12. What kind of work do you do? Do you smoke? Any alcohol use? How about recreational drugs? *(R/O HIV.)*
- ☐ 13. Now, I will be asking you some questions of a sensitive nature. I can assure you that anything you say will be kept confidential. Is that okay with you? Are you sexually active? Are your partners men, women or both? How many partners have you had during the past year? Do you use condoms? *(R/O hepatitis & AIDS.)*

Thanks for answering all these questions. At this point, I will be doing a physical examination but let me wash my hands first. *(Wash hands.)*

- ☐ 14. Can you open your mouth so I can take a look?
- ☐ 15. Now let me examine your neck for swollen glands.
- ☐ 16. Now I will be tapping your chest and belly on the right side. *(liver span)*
- ☐ 17. I will be pressing on the area below the right rib cage and let me know if it hurts. *(liver tenderness)* Now can you take a deep breath? *(liver edge)*
- ☐ 18. Now let me press the left side. Can you take a deep breath now? *(splenomegaly)*
- ☐ 19. I would like to listen to your heart.
- ☐ 20. Now, let me check for any changes on your skin.

Now let me summarize what we have talked about. You came in because of a sore throat that started ______. Based on the history and the physical examination, my initial impression of your condition is a streptococcal infection. But I am also considering other possibilities including infectious mononucleosis, diphtheria, hepatitis and the possibility of HIV infection. I will be ordering some test for more information. Do you have any questions before I go?

Challenging Questions:

HIV? That's impossible.
Where do you usually get this from?
Is this infectious?
What precautions do I need to take?
What is infectious mononucleosis?
How can I possibly have diphtheria when I have been completely immunized?
Should I stop seeing my two boyfriends?
Should I tell my roommate about it?

Sore Throat

History:

cc:	sore throat
HPI:	23 y/o WF college student c/o sore throat of 2-day duration (+) fever, (+) malaise, (+) nausea, (+) headache, (+) odynophagia; no meds taken.
PMH:	no allergies, no accidents, no injuries
FH:	parents and siblings are apparently healthy
SocH:	lives in dorm with 1 female roommate Cig (–), etoh (occasional), illicit drug use (occasional)
SexH:	sex with 2 boyfriends; uses condom every time

Physical Examination:

Gen:	A&O
VS:	T: 100° F BP: 125/85 RR: 20 cpm HR: 100 bpm
HEENT:	(+) pharyngeal and tonsillar pharyngeal erythema and edema (+) exudates, cervical lymphadenopathy no tongue enlargement nor discoloration.
Heart & Lungs:	unremarkable
Abdomen:	no hepatosplenomegaly
Skin:	no rashes

Differential Diagnosis:

1. Streptococcal infection
2. Infectious mononucleosis
3. Diphtheria
4. Hepatitis
5. HIV infection

Diagnostic Work-ups:

1. Rapid Strep & Throat culture if indicated
2. Monospot
3. CBC with differentials
4. ALT, AST, Total Bilirubin
5. HIV ELISA

CASE NO. 19

Mrs. Chanta Nguyen is a 58-year-old female who has had sudden vision loss and pain.

Vital Signs:

T **98.6° F**
P **95**
R **14**
BP **130/80**

EXPECTED TASKS

1. Gather the necessary clinical information.
2. Perform a focused and pertinent physical examination.
3. Discuss your diagnostic impressions and differential diagnosis with the patient.
4. Discuss work-ups to be ordered.
5. Complete the patient note after seeing the patient.

Vision Loss

(Knocks)

Hi, I'm Dr. ___________. How are you today? *(Shakes patient's hand.)* I'm here to examine you and ask you a few questions. By the way, do you prefer to be called Chanta or Mrs. Nguyen?

☐ 1. So, what brings you in today?
☐ 2. Did it occur suddenly or has it been going on for a long time?
☐ 3. Do you see halos around lights?
☐ 4. Have you taken any kind of medication? *(R/O steroid use.)*
☐ 5. Are they painful?
☐ 6. Any nausea and vomiting? *(R/O glaucoma.)*
☐ 7. Do you see objects better at a distance or close up?
☐ 8. Do you still see some things with this problem eye or you don't see anything at all? *(R/O cataract.)*
☐ 9. Do you use glasses or contact lenses? Since when? Do you know their grades? *(R/O refractive errors.)*
☐ 10. Can you tell me what you see when this problem occurs?
☐ 11. Is it like a veil coming down your eyes? Do you have an accompanying muscle weakness? *(R/O TIA.)*
☐ 12. Do you see flashes of lights or lights that float around? *(R/O retinal detachment.)*
☐ 13. Do you have headaches? Show me what part is most painful. *(R/O temporal arteritis.)*
☐ 14. Does it get more painful when you move your eyes? Does it feel like you're looking in a tunnel? *(R/O optic neuritis of MS.)*

- ☐ 15. Have you ever been told by a physician that you have diabetes? How about high blood pressure? Any other illness in the past? Any accidents or injuries?
- ☐ 16. I would like to ask questions about your family's health. Are you parents healthy? How about your brothers and sisters? Children?
- ☐ 17. What is your occupation? Do you drink alcohol? Do you smoke? Any use of controlled substances?
- ☐ 18. I will be asking some questions of a sensitive nature that will help me better assess your total health. I can assure you that this will all be kept confidential. Is that okay with you? Are you sexually active? Do you use any contraception? Have you ever had unprotected sex? Do you have sexual partners of the same sex, opposite sex or both? How many partners have you had during the past 12 months?

Thanks for answering all these questions. At this point, I will be doing a physical examination but let me wash my hands first. *(Wash hands.)* Would you be more comfortable if I put this drape on your legs? *(Drape patient if she answers yes.)*

- ☐ 19. I will be shining a light into your eyes. Good. Now look at my finger. Then look at the wall behind me without moving your head. Now look at this finger again. *(PERLA)*
- ☐ 20. Follow my finger with your eyes without moving your head. *(EOM)*
- ☐ 21. I will be looking into your eyes with this instrument. Let me dim the lights so I can better see it. Now, just look straight ahead while I do this. *(Funduscopy)*
- ☐ 22. I will be listening to some sounds on your neck. *(Carotid bruit)*
- ☐ 23. I will be checking your tummy.
- ☐ 24. I will do some tests on your arms and legs. *(Motor, DTR, sensory)*

Now let me summarize what we have talked about. You came because of a vision loss. Based on the history and the physical examination my initial impression of your condition is a glaucoma, but I am also considering other possibilities including cataract, refractive errors, TIA, and temporal arteritis. Therefore, I will be ordering some tests to make sure we're on the right track. Do you have any questions before I go?

Challenging Questions:

What is TIA?
What causes glaucoma?
What causes cataracts?
Is this just a problem of incorrect glasses?
What is temporal arteritis?
What tests are you ordering?
Am I going blind?
I think you should refer me to an eye specialist.
Is this related to aging?

Vision Loss

History

cc:	vision loss
HPI:	– 58 y/o Asian female c/o sudden vision loss with pain
	– Started 2 hrs ago after coming out of the theater
	– (+) halo around lights; no nausea, no vomiting
	– uses eyeglasses only for reading; no flashes or floaters;
	– no veil-like vision loss; no tunnel vision
	– slightly painful when eyes are moved
	– not taking any medications
	– (+) generalized abdominal pain
PMH:	no allergies, no accidents, no injuries
FamH:	father had CHF; mother had epilepsy
SocH:	works as a cytotechnologist
	cig (–), etoh (on social gatherings only), illicit drugs (–)
SexH:	sex with husband only
OB/GYN:	G3P3

Physical Examination:

Gen:	A&O X3; in acute distress
VS:	WNL except BP 130/80
HEENT:	(+) red eyes B/L; steamy cornea
	dilated pupil not reactive to light
	globe hard on palpation
Abd:	NABS, (+) generalized tenderness
Neuro:	DTR ++ X4, sensory intact X4, motor 5/5 X4

Differential Diagnosis:

1. Glaucoma
2. Cataract
3. Refractive errors
4. TIA
5. Temporal Arteritis

Diagnostic Work-ups:

1. Tonometry
2. Snellen's Chart
3. Doppler of the carotid arteries
4. ESR
5. FBS

CASE NO. 20

Mr. William Collins is a 66-year-old male who came in complaining of hearing loss.

Vital Signs:

T 98.4° F
P 72
R 17
BP 125/80

EXPECTED TASKS

1. Gather the necessary clinical information.
2. Perform a focused and pertinent physical examination.
3. Discuss your diagnostic impressions and differential diagnosis with the patient.
4. Discuss work-ups to be ordered.
5. Complete the patient note after seeing the patient.

Hearing Loss

(Knocks)

Hi, I'm Dr. ________. How are you today? *(Shakes patient's hand.)* I'm here to examine you and ask you a few questions. By the way, do you prefer to be called William, Bill or Mr. Collins?

- ☐ 1. So, what brings you in today?
  (Mnemonic: MNOPQRST)
- ☐ 2. **M**edications: Are you taking any medication right now? Antibiotics? Diuretics?
- ☐ 3. **N**oise Exposure: Have you ever had constant exposure to a noisy environment?
- ☐ 4. **O**nset: When did it start?
- ☐ 5. **P**ain: Do you have any pain in your ear?
- ☐ 6. **P**artial or Complete: Do you hear something with this ear or nothing at all?
- ☐ 7. **Q**ueasy feeling: Do you feel queasy or nauseous? Any vomiting? Any feeling of being spun around?
- ☐ 8. **R**ecent infection: Any recent infection I should know about?
- ☐ 9. **S**ide: What side gives you more difficulty in hearing?
- ☐ 10. **T**innitus: Do you hear any ringing in your ear?
- ☐ 11. **T**rauma: Any history of accident or injury that could have caused this?

- ☐ 12. Have you had any illnesses in the past? Any accidents or allergies?
- ☐ 13. I will be asking you about diseases in the family, OK? Are your parents still healthy? How about your brothers and sisters? How about your wife and children?
- ☐ 14. What kind of work do you do? Do you use any recreational drugs?

- ☐ 15. Now, I will be asking you some questions of a sensitive nature. I can assure you that anything you say will be kept confidential. I need to ask these questions so I can have a clearer picture of your overall health status. Are you sexually active? Are your partners men, women or both? How many partners have you had during the past year? Do you use condoms?

Thanks for answering all these questions At this point, I will be doing a physical examination but let me wash my hands first. *(Wash hands.)* Would you be more comfortable if I put this drape on your legs? *(Drape patient if he answers yes.)*

- ☐ 16. I will be closing your other ear and whisper some numbers in this ear. I'd like you to repeat each number that I say.
- ☐ 17. Let me look in your ear with this instrument. *(Otoscopy)*
- ☐ 18. I will be placing this instrument on your forehead. Tell me if you hear the sound to the right, left or middle. *(Weber test)*
- ☐ 19. Now, I will be placing this instrument behind your ear and let me know if you don't hear the sound anymore. After that, I will transfer this instrument in front of your ear and let me know if you no longer hear the sound. *(Rinne test)*
- ☐ 20. I will be checking your heart and lungs.

Now let me summarize what we have talked about. You came because of a hearing difficulty that started five years ago and has progressively worsened. Based on the history and the physical examination my initial impression of your condition is presbycusis which is a hearing loss due to aging. But I am also considering other possibilities including medication toxicity, Diabetes mellitus, acoustic neuroma and Meniere's Disease. I will be ordering some tests to make sure that we consider all the possible scenarios so we can make a better decision on how we will deal with your condition. Do you have any question before I go?

(If it is a conductive hearing loss, consider cerumen impaction, foreign body, otitis externa or perforated tympanic membrane. If it is a sensori-neural case, consider presbycusis, drug toxicity, acoustic neuroma, Meniere's Disease, and Diabetes mellitus.)

Challenging Questions:

Is this related to aging?
What is Meniere's Disease?
I think this is due to my previous job as a construction worker. Do you agree, Doc?
I think I should sue the company I used to work for.
Should I start wearing a hearing aid?
Are you saying I have diabetes?
Can diabetes cause hearing loss?
What causes acoustic neuroma?

Hearing Loss

History:

cc:	hearing loss
HPI:	66 y/o WM c/o progressive hearing loss of 5-yr duration – now retired but worked as a road construction worker for 35 years – h/o taking an "antibiotic" for a lung infection several months ago – no fever, no nausea, no vomiting – no vertigo, no tinnitus, no ear discharge
PMH:	car accident at 24 y/o; cholecystectomy at 40 y/o
FamH:	both parents were diabetic
SocH:	etoh occasional, cig 20 ppd but stopped 5 yrs ago, no illicit drug use
Sex:	sexually active with wife only

Physical Examination:

Gen:	A&O X3
VS:	WNL
HEENT:	external auditory canal has no erythema, edema or discharge – ear tenderness (–); tympanic membrane unremarkable – no foreign body or impacted cerumen seen – no postauricular pain – (+) difficulty in hearing whispered word on the right side – Weber: lateralizes to the left – Rinne: AC>BC
Lungs:	symmetrical; wheezing (+) B/L, no rales, no dullness, normal vocal and tactile fremitus

Differential Diagnosis:

1. Presbycusis
2. Drug toxicity
3. Diabetes mellitus
4. Acoustic neuroma
5. Meniere's Disease

Diagnostic Work-ups:

1. Audiology exam
2. Drug level (specific drug, e.g. gentamicin or other aminoglycosides)
3. Tympanometry
4. FBS
5. MRI

CASE NO. 21

Brenda Friedman is a 33-year-old female patient wants to see you today because of ear pain.

Vital Signs:

T 100.2° F
P 101
R 22
BP 115/70

EXPECTED TASKS

1. Gather the necessary clinical information.
2. Perform a focused and pertinent physical examination.
3. Discuss your diagnostic impressions and differential diagnosis with the patient.
4. Discuss work-ups to be ordered.
5. Complete the patient note after seeing the patient.

Ear Pain

(Knocks)

Hi, I'm Dr. ________. How are you today? *(Shakes patient's hand.)* I'm here to examine you today and ask you a few questions. By the way, do you prefer to be called Brenda or Ms. Friedman?

- ☐ 1. So, what brings you in today?
- ☐ 2. When did this start?
- ☐ 3. Have you noticed any discharge coming out of your ear? What does it look like? How does it smell? Any changes in your hearing? *(Otitis media)*
- ☐ 4. How often do you swim?
- ☐ 5. Do you have diabetes? *(Otitis externa)*
- ☐ 6. Do you have a sore throat? How about difficulty in swallowing? Any fever? *(Tonsilitis)*
- ☐ 7. Do you hear a clicking sound in your jaw when you yawn or open your mouth? Any pain when you chew your food? *(TMJ problems)*
- ☐ 8. Have you had any illnesses in the past? Any accidents or allergies?
- ☐ 9. I will be asking you about diseases in the family, OK? Are your parents healthy? How about your brothers and sisters? How about your husband and children?
- ☐ 10. What kind of work do you do? Do you use any recreational drugs?
- ☐ 11. Now, I will be asking you some questions of a sensitive nature. I can assure you that anything you say will be kept confidential. Your answers will help give me a clearer picture of your overall health. Are you sexually active? Are your partners men, women or both? How many partners have you had during the past year? Do you use condoms?

Thanks for answering all these questions. At this point, I will be doing a physical examination but let me wash my hands first. *(Wash hands.)* Would you be more comfortable if I put this drape on your legs? *(Drape patient if she answers yes.)*

- ☐ 12. I would like to take a look inside your ear with this instrument. *(Otoscopy)*
- ☐ 13. I will be pulling your ear. Let me know if you feel any pain when I do it. *(R/O Otitis externa.)*
- ☐ 14. Can you open your mouth? I want to take a look at your throat.
- ☐ 15. I will be touching the joint in front of your ear now. Can you open your mouth while I do this? *(R/O TMJ.)*
- ☐ 16. I will be pressing on the tiny bumps behind your ears. Let me know if you feel any pain. *(R/O Mastoiditis.)*
- ☐ 17. I will be checking your neck. *(Check for lymphadenopathy.)*

Now, let me summarize what we have talked about. You came in because of this ear pain that started a couple of days ago. Based on the history and the physical examination my initial impression of your condition is what is called otitis externa, but I am also considering other possibilities including otitis media, tonsillitis, mastoiditis, and an impacted cerumen or foreign body in the ear. I will be ordering some tests to make sure that we consider all the possible scenarios. Do you have any questions before I go?

Challenging Questions:

What is otitis?
What is a cerumen?
Is mastoiditis infectious?
How can tonsilitis cause hearing problems?
Am I gonna go deaf?
What tests are you ordering?
Do you think my insurance will cover these tests?

Ear Pain

History

cc:	ear pain
HPI:	33 y/o WF c/o progressive ear pain of 2 days duration
	h/o swimming 8 days ago
	(+) itching, (+) fever, (–) discharge
	no nausea, no vomiting
	pain worsened by touching the ear
	no pain during mastication
	no meds taken

PMH:	no h/o hospitalization except for childbirth
FamH:	father had diabetes, mother has rheumatoid arthritis
SocH:	etoh (–), cig (–), illicit drug (–)
SexH:	sexually active with husband only
OB/GYN:	G2P2

Physical Examination

Gen:	A&O X3
VS:	T: 100.2° F P: 101 R: 22 BP: 115/70
HEENT:	(+) erythema & edema of the external auditory canal (+) ear tenderness; unremarkable tympanic membranes no post auricular pain; no foreign body seen pharynx and tonsils unremarkable no neck lymphadenopathy

Differential Diagnosis:

1. Otitis externa
2. Otitis media
3. Tonsilitis
4. Mastoiditis
5. Cerumen or foreign body in the ear

Diagnostic Work-ups:

1. Tympanometry
2. Swab for C&S
3. FBS
4. CBC with diff
5. CT or MRI

CASE NO. 22

Mrs. Nancy Adams is a 71-year-old female complaining of forgetfulness.

Vital Signs:

T 98.5° F
P 90
R 14
BP 135/85

EXPECTED TASKS

1. Gather the necessary clinical information.
2. Perform a focused and pertinent physical examination.
3. Discuss your diagnostic impressions and differential diagnosis with the patient.
4. Discuss work-ups to be ordered.
5. Complete the patient note after seeing the patient.

Forgetfulness (Alzheimer's Disease)

(Knocks)

Hi, I'm Dr. ________ and I'm here to examine you today. Do you prefer to be called Mrs. Adams or Nancy?

- ☐ 1. So, what brings you in today? *(HPI)*
- ☐ 2. Have you ever been hospitalized before? How about accidents or injuries? *(PMH)*
- ☐ 3. Are you taking any medication right now? How about in the past? *(PMH)*
- ☐ 4. Now, I'd like to know something about your family's health. Has anyone in your immediate family — parents, brothers, sisters and children — ever had surgery or specific illnesses that you can think of? *(FamH)*
- ☐ 5. Any family member with problems concentrating or thinking clearly? Depression? Thyroid problems? *(FamH)*
- ☐ 6. What is your occupation? Any history of tobacco use? How about alcohol? Recreational drugs? *(SocH)*
- ☐ 7. Now I will be asking you questions of a sensitive nature but is important in making a good assessment of your condition. Are you still sexually active? *(SexH)*
- ☐ 8. Who do you live with? Do you feel safe at home? Do you have somebody you can turn to when you have problems? *(R/O abuse.)*
- ☐ 9. Do you have any trouble dressing? How about eating, walking around or going to the bathroom? *(ADL)*
- ☐ 10. Who does your shopping? How do you keep up with daily house chores and bills? *(IADL)*

- ☐ 11. How would you describe your mood? Have you noticed any changes in your interests? Do you sleep well? Have you ever had thoughts of hurting yourself or other people? *(R/O depression.)*
- ☐ 12. Have you noticed any changes in your weight? How's your appetite? Do you feel bothered more by hot or cold temperature? *(R/O Hypothyroidism.)*

At this point, I will be asking you some more questions and do some things which will give me an idea of your total health.

- ☐ 13. Where are you right now? Do you know today's date? Who am I? *(Orientation)*
- ☐ 14. What did you have for breakfast this morning? Who was the president of the United States before Ronald Reagan? *(Memory)*
- ☐ 15. What do you get if you subtract 7 from 100? Subtract seven again from the result? *(Attention/Math)*
- ☐ 16. Do you ever feel like you are seeing things that other people don't see? *(Visual Hallucination)* Do you ever feel like you are hearing things that others don't hear? *(Auditory Hallucination)* Have you ever been told that you have very unrealistic goals for yourself? *(Delusion)*
- ☐ 17. What would you do if you saw a $10 bill on the sidewalk? *(Judgment)*

Now, I am going to do a physical exam on you but let me wash my hands first. *(Wash hands.)* Let me put this drape on so you'll feel more comfortable. *(Drape patient.)*

- ☐ 18. I will be checking your thyroid. *(palpate thyroid)* Can you put your chin down and slightly to the right? I will be pressing on this side *(displace larynx to the right side)* and I will ask you to swallow while I check your thyroid. OK, now swallow. Good. Now let's do it on the other side.
- ☐ 19. I will be listening to your neck. *(Carotid Bruits)*
- ☐ 20. I would like to listen to your heart.
- ☐ 21. Can you push your arms/forearms/hands upward against my hand? Now let's do it downward.
- ☐ 22. I will now check the reflexes in your arms. I will now check the reflexes in your legs.
- ☐ 23. Can you push your thighs/legs/feet upward against my hand? Now let's do it downward.
- ☐ 24. Can you get up and walk across the room and back?
- ☐ 25. I will be checking your nerves. *(Do cranial nerve tests from CN3 to CN12.)*

Now, Mrs. Adams, I would like to summarize what you've told me. You said that you've become forgetful and this seemed to get worse and worse. You also said that ______. My initial impression of your condition is dementia of the Alzheimer's type — in other words, forgetfulness due to some changes occurring in the brain. I am also considering other possibilities including major depression, hypothyroidism, multi-infarct dementia and Vit B_{12} deficiency. That is why I am ordering some tests which include different blood tests and a CT scan of the head. So, do you have any questions before I go?

Challenging Questions:

What? I'm sorry I wasn't paying too much attention.
Alzheimer's? I think I'm better off dead.
Those are very expensive tests, Doc. Will Medicare pay for them?
What causes Alzheimer's Disease?
Do you honestly think I am going insane?
How many more years do I have?
How can this happen? I take my vitamins every day.
Do you think I should start taking *Ginko biloba*?

Forgetfulness (Alzheimer's Disease)

History:

cc:	forgetfulness
HPI:	71 y/o WF c/o forgetfulness ADLs impaired. IADLs impaired (+) lack of energy and reduced concentration, (–) tremors at rest (–) suicidal or homicidal ideation (–) intolerance to cold
PMH:	no h/o medical use including "mood medications"
FamH:	significant for DM and heart disease
SocH:	cig (–), etoh (–); lives in a nursing home

Physical Examination:

VS:	WNL except BP 135/85
Neck:	thyroid has no tenderness, no nodules, no enlargement, no mass
Neuro:	slow speech but no shuffling gait or bradykinesia CN III-XII intact motor strength: 5/5 X4 extremities sensation: intact
DTRs:	++ X4 extremities
CV:	NRRR, PMI not displaced ; no murmurs, gallops, rubs or clicks
MMSE:	A&O X2; speech is slow but goal-directed; recent memory is intact; remote memory is impaired; concentration is impaired as tested by serial sevens; mood is depressed and consistent with affect; no abnormal perceptions; no suicidal or homicidal ideation; judgment is impaired.

Differential Diagnosis:

1. Dementia (Alzheimer's type)
2. Major Depression
3. Hypothyroidism
4. Multi-infarct Dementia
5. Vit B12 Deficiency

Diagnostic Work-ups:

1. TSH/T3/FT4
2. CT scan of the head
3. CBC
4. Serum B12 level
5. Carotid duplex Doppler scanning

CASE NO. 23

Mr. Eric Fisher is a 70-year-old male who came in with difficulty of urination.

Vital Signs:

T 98°F
P 70
R 16
BP 130/80

EXPECTED TASKS

1. Gather the necessary clinical information.
2. Perform a focused and pertinent physical examination.
3. Discuss your diagnostic impressions and differential diagnosis with the patient.
4. Discuss work-ups to be ordered.
5. Complete the patient note after seeing the patient.

Difficulty of Urination

(Knocks)

Hi, I'm Dr. __________ and I'm here to examine you today. So, Mr. Fisher, what brings you in today?

☐ 1. Do you have any trouble peeing?
☐ 2. Does it burn when you pee?
☐ 3. Are you peeing more frequently than usual?
☐ 4. How often do you pee at night?
☐ 5. Do you notice any color changes in your urine?
☐ 6. Do you have any problem starting your urine?
☐ 7. Do you have any problem stopping your urine?
☐ 8. Does your urine leak when you cough or sneeze?
☐ 9. Do you feel like you need to use the bathroom in a hurry?
☐ 10. Have you noticed any change in the size or force of the stream?
☐ 11. Do you feel like there is urine left in your bladder after you pee?
☐ 12. Have you been hospitalized before? Any history of accidents or injuries?
☐ 13. Are your parents alive? How about your wife? How's her health? How about your kids? How's their health?
☐ 14. Do you still work? What was your job before? Do you drink alcoholic beverages? Do you smoke? Have you ever used any recreational drugs?
☐ 15. I usually ask questions about sexual habits as part of my routine evaluation. You can be assured that everything will be kept confidential. Is that okay with you? All right, then. Are you are sexually active? Do you use any contraception? Have you ever had unprotected sex? Do you have sexual partners of the same sex, opposite sex or both? How many partners have you had during the past 12 months?

We have reviewed a lot of information. Now, I will be doing a physical examination but let me wash my hands first. *(Wash hands.)* Would you be more comfortable if I put this drape on your legs? *(Drape patient if he says yes.)*

☐ 16. Let me listen to your chest.
☐ 17. I will be checking your belly. *(Include CVA tenderness.)*
☐ 18. I will be doing some tests on your legs. *(Do motor, sensory and DTR.)*

Now, I would like to summarize what you've told me. You said that ______. You also said that… My initial impression of your condition is benign prostatic hyperplasia. This is a kind of condition where your prostate becomes more active than normal. But I am also considering some other possibilities including cancer of the prostate, nephrolithiasis or kidney stones, prostatitis or inflammation of the prostate, and cancer of the lungs. That is why I am ordering some tests which include a rectal exam, a genital exam, PSA, a urine test, and x-rays of the chest and abdomen. Do you have any questions before I leave?

Challenging Questions:

What are the odds that this is cancer?
I am calling my children to tell them I have cancer.
What is the normal PSA?
Can you give me an estimate on how much longer will I live?
If I'm going to die, I wanna die at home—not in the hospital.
What caused this?
I do not want to wear any adult diapers.
Am I gonna have an operation?

Difficulty of Urination

cc:	difficulty of urination
HPI:	70 y/o male c/o difficulty of urination that started 1–2 mos. ago. dribbling (+), straining (+), feeling residual urine (+), urgency (+) nocturia (–), hematuria (–), incontinence (–), dysuria (–), fever (–). decreased size and force of stream. increased frequency of urination since the problem started. only taking vitamins and cholesterol-lowering drugs. No other meds being taken.
PMH:	no h/o kidney disease had surgery for lung CA 20 years ago no accidents or allergies
FH:	no kidney disease
SocH:	retired teacher, etoh (–) since 3 years ago, cig (–) for the last 25 years, recreational drugs (–).
SexH:	no h/o STD, no sexual intercourse since 2 years ago.

Physical Examination:

Gen:	A&O; not in acute pain or distress
VS:	WNL except BP 130/80
Lungs:	symmetrical; no wheezing B/L; no rales, no dullness; N vocal & tactile fremitus
Abdomen:	NABS, tympanitic on percussion, no tenderness on light and deep palpation X4 quadrants; CVA tenderness (–). Neuro: motor strength on lower extremities (5/5) DTRs (2+) and intact sensation B/L on lower extremities

Differential Diagnosis:

1. Benign Prostatic Hyperplasia (Hypertrophy)
2. Prostatic CA
3. Nephrolithiasis
4. Prostatitis
5. Lung CA (possibly metastatic)

Diagnostic Work-ups:

1. Rectal and Genital Exam
2. PSA
3. Urinalysis, C&S if indicated
4. Abdominal X-ray
5. Chest X-ray

CASE NO. 24

Mr. Dennis Thompson is a 20-year-old African-American male who came in for prescription refill for his shoulder pain.

Vital Signs:

T 98°F
P 75
R 14
BP 135/90

EXPECTED TASKS

1. Gather the necessary clinical information.
2. Perform a focused and pertinent physical examination.
3. Discuss your diagnostic impressions and differential diagnosis with the patient.
4. Discuss work-ups to be ordered.
5. Complete the patient note after seeing the patient.

Substance Abuse

(Knocks)

Hi, Mr. Thompson, I'm Dr. ______ and I'm here to examine you today.

☐ 1. So, what brings you in today?
(Mnemonic: LMNOPQRST)
☐ 2. **L**ocation: Can you tell me exactly where the pain is?
☐ 3. **M**edications: Have you taken any medications for it?
☐ 4. **N** & V and other symptoms: Do you have nausea? Vomiting? Fever?
☐ 5. **O**nset: When did it start? Have you had trauma in this area?
☐ 6. **P**recipitating factor: What makes it worse?
☐ 7. **Q**uality: How would you describe the pain?
☐ 8. **R**adiation/**R**elieving Factors: Does it go anywhere? What makes it better?
☐ 9. **S**everity: On a scale of 1–10 where ten is the most painful, where will you rank this pain?
☐ 10. **T**iming: What particular time of the day does the pain occur?

(Patient will continue talking about his need for pain relief and may even make a suggestion as to which pain medication works best for him. Answer him like this: *"I know you are having problems but I need to ask you a few more questions so I can make a better assessment of your condition."*)

☐ 11. Have you had any accidents or injuries in the past? Any illnesses in the past? How about allergies?
☐ 12. How are your parents' health? How about your spouse? How about your brothers and sisters? Do you have kids? How's their health?

☐ 13. What type of job do you do? Is it stressful? Are you engaged in sports? Do you drink alcoholic beverages? (If patient answers yes, ask CAGE question~**C**ut, **A**nnoyed, **G**uilty, **E**ye opener) Do you smoke? Any use of recreational drugs? (Patient would say "*yes*" or "*occasionally*") How often?

☐ 14. I usually ask questions about sexual habits as part of my routine evaluation. You can be assured that everything you say will be kept confidential. Is that okay with you? All right, then. Are you are sexually active? Do you use any contraception? Have you ever had unprotected sex? Do you have sexual partners of the same sex, opposite sex or both? How many partners have you had during the past 12 months?

We have reviewed a lot of information. Now, I will be doing a physical examination but let me wash my hands first. *(Wash hands.)* Would you be more comfortable if I put this drape on your legs? *(Drape patient if he says yes.)*

☐ 15. I will be moving your shoulder. *(Range of motion: R/O rotator cuff tear which is pain with shoulder shrug on arm abduction; R/O bicipital tendonitis which is shoulder pain when the forearm is supinated against resistance; R/O tricipital tendonitis which is pain in the triceps areas when the forearm is supinated against resistance.)*

☐ 16. I will be pressing on your shoulder joint. *(Note any swelling, asymmetry or deformities.)*

☐ 17. Let's check your reflexes now. *(Do biceps, triceps.)*

☐ 18. I will be checking the sensation on your arms. *(Sensory)*

☐ 19. Can you open your hand while I grab your fingers? *(Motor)*

(Important: when checking joints, always test the other side or do both simultaneously if possible; also check the joint above and below it).

Now let me summarize what you've told me. You said you have pain that affects your right shoulder and you feel that only Demerol gives you relief. Considering everything you've told me, I have a feeling that the bigger issue here is your dependence on pain killers. But I also want to find out how serious your shoulder problem is, so I am ordering several tests to make sure we are on the right track. Do you have any questions?

Challenging Questions:

I've tried other pain killers, but only Demerol gives me relief.
I'm not a drug addict.
Can you just give me the damn thing!
You've got to help me.
I need this medicine so I can get back to work.

Substance Abuse

History:

cc:	prescription refill request
HPI:	20 y/o AAM requesting a refill for Demerol. Was seen in ER 2 mos ago for abdominal pain. Also c/o of dull R shoulder pain that that keeps recurring Cig (+) 3 sticks/day for the past 2 yrs.; etoh (+) occasionally; recreational drugs (+) Unemployed, lives with parents Plays basketball every other day but no h/o trauma in the shoulder. Occasional sex with 2 girlfriends without using condoms

Physical Examination

Gen:	A&O
VS:	WNL except BP 135/90
Shoulder Joints & Upper Extremities:	ROM not limited, intact sensation, motor 5/5, reflex ++
Skin:	no needle track marks

Differential Diagnosis:

1. Substance abuse
2. Rotator cuff tear
3. Sickle cell disease
4. Tendinitis
5. Malingering

Diagnostic Work-ups:

1. Urine drug screen
2. X-ray of the shoulder joint
3. Sickle screen
4. CBC with diff
5. HIV ELISA

CASE NO. 25

Mr. Enrique Vasquez is a 42-year-old male complaining of a 25-lb weight loss in the past two months.

Vital Signs:

T 99.2° F
P 70
R 14
BP 125/75

EXPECTED TASKS

1. Gather the necessary clinical information.
2. Perform a focused and pertinent physical examination.
3. Discuss your diagnostic impressions and differential diagnosis with the patient.
4. Discuss work-ups to be ordered.
5. Complete the patient note after seeing the patient.

HIV

(Knocks)

Hi, I'm Dr. __________ and I'm here to examine you today. Do you prefer to be called Mr. Vasquez or Enrique?

- ☐ 1. So, what brings you in today?
- ☐ 2. When did it start? How much weight have you lost?
- ☐ 3. Any other changes you have noticed recently?
- ☐ 4. You said afternoon fever. Do you use a thermometer?
- ☐ 5. Any cough? Does it produce any gunk? What color? How often does this happen?
- ☐ 6. Any changes in your bowel habits? How often do you have diarrhea? Do you see blood in your stool?
- ☐ 7 Have you ever been hospitalized before? Any accidents or injuries? Allergies? Any similar episodes of headache before?
- ☐ 8. Are your parents living? How's their health? How about your brothers and sisters? Do you have children? How's their health? Any history of asthma?
- ☐ 9. What is your occupation? Do you feel stressed at work? Do you use tobacco products? For how long? How about alcohol? Do you take any kind of recreational drugs? Who do you live with?
- ☐ 10. I will be asking some questions of a sensitive nature that will help me better assess your total health. I can assure you that this will all be kept confidential. Is that okay with you? Are you sexually active? Do you use any contraception? Have you ever had unprotected sex? Do you have sexual partners of the same sex, opposite sex or both? How many partners have you had during the past 12 months?

Thanks for answering these questions. Now I will be examining some parts of your body but let me wash my hands first. *(Wash hands.)*

- ☐ 11. Can you open your mouth and say "Ah-"?
- ☐ 12. I will feel your neck, armpits and groin for bumps or lumps.
- ☐ 13. I will be examining your chest.
- ☐ 14. Now, can you say "99" while I listen to your chest? Do that once again while I move my hands on various areas of your chest and back. *(Fremitus)*
- ☐ 15. I will be tapping on your chest.
- ☐ 16. I will be listening to your lungs. Breathe in and breathe out.
- ☐ 17. I will be examining your belly.

Now let me summarize what you've told me. You said you have a weight loss of 25 lbs in the past 2 months. You also complained of occasional diarrhea and slight fever in the afternoon. Based on this, plus some other personal information that you have provided me, my initial impression is HIV infection. There are also other diseases that have the same symptoms, including TB, cancer, hyperthyroidism, and substance abuse, so I will be ordering some lab work for more information. Once we get the results back, we can discuss the results of these exams. Do you have any questions?

Challenging Questions:

If my HIV test comes back positive, how long will I live?
How can I get TB when I have not been exposed to anybody with TB?
How long will it take to get the HIV result?
Am I going to die?
Should I tell my partner?
What precautions should I take?

HIV

History:

cc:	weight loss
HPI:	42 y/o Hispanic male c/o weight loss (25 lbs) for the last 2 mos. He has occasional episodes of diarrhea but no constipation. He has slight fever in the afternoon but no cough or chest pain. He works as a lawyer and admits to having homosexual unprotected sex. Cig (–), etoh occasionally, drugs (–). His family and past medical history are unremarkable.

Physical Examination:

Gen:	A&O X3, cooperative, not in distress
VS:	WNL except for T 99.2° F
HEENT:	no oral cavity lesions; no neck or postauricular lymphadenopathy
Lungs:	N breath sounds, no rales, N tactile and vocal fremitus
Abdomen:	N ABS, no tenderness, no organomegaly
Skin:	no lesions

Differential Diagnosis:

1. HIV infection
2. Pulmonary TB
3. Malignancy
4. Hyperthyroidism
5. Substance Abuse

Diagnostic Work-ups:

1. HIV ELISA
2. CXR
3. FOBT
4. TSH/FT4
5. Urine Drug Screen

CASE NO. 26

Ms. Elizabeth Patel is a 40-year-old Asian female who has palpitations.

Vital Signs:

T 98.3
P 101
R 16
BP 130/90

EXPECTED TASKS

1. Gather the necessary clinical information.
2. Perform a focused and pertinent physical examination.
3. Discuss your diagnostic impressions and differential diagnosis with the patient.
4. Discuss work-ups to be ordered.
5. Complete the patient note after seeing the patient.

Palpitations

(Knocks)

Hi, I'm Dr. _______ and I'm here to examine you today. Do you prefer to be called Ms. Patel or Elizabeth?

- ☐ 1. So, what brings you in today?
- ☐ 2. Onset: When did it start?
- ☐ 3. Do you have any trouble chewing or swallowing?
- ☐ 4. Do you have trouble adjusting to the temperature in a room? Do you prefer it warm or cold?
- ☐ 5. How's your appetite?
- ☐ 6. Have you noticed any weight changes lately?
- ☐ 7. Do you feel like you are thirsty all the time?
- ☐ 8. Do you feel like you want to pee all the time?
- ☐ 9. Have you noticed any changes in your hair recently?
- ☐ 10. Have you noticed any changes in the size of your shoes or hat?
- ☐ 11. How would you describe your mood?
- ☐ 12. When was the last time you had a blood count? What was the result?
- ☐ 13. Have you ever been hospitalized before? Any accidents or injuries? Allergies?
- ☐ 14. Are your parents living? How's their health? How about your brothers and sisters? Do you have children? How's their health?
- ☐ 15. What is your occupation? Do you feel stressed at work? Do you use tobacco products? For how long? How about alcohol? Do you take any kind of recreational drugs? Who do you live with?

☐ 16. I will be asking some questions of a sensitive nature that will help me better assess your total health. I can assure you that this will all be kept confidential. Is that okay with you? Are you sexually active? Do you use any contraception? Have you ever had unprotected sex? Do you have sexual partners of the same sex, opposite sex or both? How many partners have you had during the past 12 months?

Thank you for answering all those questions. Now, I will be doing a physical examination but let me wash my hands first. *(Wash hands.)* Would you be more comfortable if I put this drape on your legs? *(Drape patient if she says yes.)*

☐ 17. I will be checking your eyes. *(pallor for lid lag)*
☐ 18. I will be shining this light on your eyes. Just look straight while I do this. *(funduscopic to R/O DM changes)*
☐ 19. I will be examining your thyroid. *(Palpate thyroid)*
☐ 20. Can you put your chin down and slightly to the right? I will be pressing on this side *(displace larynx to the right side)* and I will ask you to swallow while I feel your thyroid. OK, now swallow. Good. Now let's do it on the other side.
☐ 21. I will be listening to your neck. *(Carotid bruits)*
☐ 22. I would like to listen to your heart and lungs.
☐ 23. I will be checking your muscle strength and reflexes.

Now let me summarize what we have talked about. You came because of palpitations which was accompanied by a weight loss of eight pounds. Based on the history and the physical examination my initial impression of your condition is hyperthyroidism. But I am also considering other possibilities like anemia, mitral valve prolapse, arrhythmia, and substance abuse. I will be ordering some tests to make sure that we consider all the possible scenarios so we can make better decisions on how we will deal with your condition. Do you have any question before I go?

Challenging Questions:

Is this the same as goiter?
If this is a thyroid problem, how come my neck doesn't appear swollen?
Should I start taking iron pills?
You mean, I have heart problems?
What is the possibility of a heart attack?
I am very nervous, Doc.
I don't use drugs.

Palpitations

History:

cc:	palpitations
HPI:	– 40 y/o Asian F c/o palpitations
	– started 7 days ago usually occurring at no specific time of the day
	– weight loss of 8 lbs since 6 mos ago
	– normal appetite
	– bothered by hot weather
	– feels tired all the time
	– sleeps about 5 hrs/day
	– no diarrhea or constipation noted
PMH:	PUD diagnosed 4 years ago; cured as claimed
FamH:	father has hypertension; mother has kidney problems
SocH:	works as a secretary; job considered not stressful
	cig (–), etoh (–), drugs of abuse (–)
	sexually active with husband only

Physical examination:

Gen:	well-groomed, not in distress
VS:	WNL except HR 101 & BP 130/90
HEENT:	no lid lag
Neck:	thyroid not enlarged; no nodules; no tenderness
Neuro:	motor 5/5 X4; DTR ++ X4
Heart:	no murmurs, PMI not displaced, no JVD, no pedal edema, no cyanosis
Lungs:	unremarkable

Differential Diagnosis:

1. Hyperthyroidism
2. Anemia
3. MVP
4. Arrhythmia
5. Substance Abuse (Cocaine, caffeine)

Diagnostic Work-ups:

1. TSH
2. CBC
3. Echocardiography
4. ECG/Holter monitoring
5. Urine Drug Screen

CASE NO. 27

Mrs. Joan Turner is a 48-year-old female who complains of "paleness."

Vital Signs:

T 98° F
P 98
R 14
BP 120/80

EXPECTED TASKS

1. Gather the necessary clinical information.
2. Perform a focused and pertinent physical examination.
3. Discuss your diagnostic impressions and differential diagnosis with the patient.
4. Discuss work-ups to be ordered.
5. Complete the patient note after seeing the patient.

Pallor

(Knocks)

Hi, I'm Dr. _______ and I'm here to examine you today. Do you prefer to be called Mrs.Turner or Joan?

- ☐ 1. So, what brings you in today?
- ☐ 2. When did it start?
- ☐ 3. When was the last time you had a blood count? What was the result?
- ☐ 4. Do you bleed or bruise easily? Any nose bleeds?
- ☐ 5. Are you taking any medication right now?
- ☐ 6. Are you taking any vitamins? What kind?
- ☐ 7. Have you lost any weight recently?
- ☐ 8. Any change in bowel habits?
- ☐ 9. What is the usual color of your stool?
- ☐ 10. How's your appetite?
- ☐ 11. Any nausea or vomiting? Any fever?
- ☐ 12. Is your period regular each month? How long do they last? How many pads/tampons do you use per day? Are they mildly, moderately or fully soaked?
- ☐ 13. Have you ever been hospitalized before? Any accidents or injuries? Allergies?
- ☐ 14. Are your parents living? How's their health? How about your brothers and sisters? Do you have children? How's their health? Any family member with a bleeding disorder?
- ☐ 15. What is your occupation? Do you feel stressed at work? Do you use tobacco products? For how long? How about alcohol? Do you take any kind of recreational drugs? Who do you live with?

☐ 16. I will be asking some questions of a sensitive nature that will help me better assess your total health. I can assure you that this will all be kept confidential. Is that okay with you? Are you sexually active? Do you use any contraception? Have you ever had unprotected sex? Do you have sexual partners of the same sex, opposite sex or both? How many partners have you had during the past 12 months?

Now, I will do a physical exam. Let me wash my hands first. *(Wash hands)*. Let me put this drape on you so you will feel more comfortable.

☐ 17. Let me take a look at your eyes and your eyelids.
☐ 18. Let me look at your fingernails.
☐ 19. I will be examining your belly. *(inspection, auscultation, palpation, percussion)*

Now let me summarize what we have talked about. You came because of paleness accompanied by nausea. Based on the history and the physical examination my initial impression of your condition is iron deficiency anemia. Other possibilities include pernicious anemia, thallasemia, a tumor in the food passages and leukemia. I will be ordering some lab tests and once we get the results back we will discuss what treatment options we have. Do you have any questions before I leave?

Challenging Questions:

Leukemia? That sounds scary.
What is thallasemia?
Do I have cancer?
What is pernicious anemia?
Is this something genetic?
Why do I look pale? I take vitamins everyday.
What is a CBC?

Pallor

History:

cc:	Pallor
HPI:	48-y/o WF c/o "paleness" for 1 mo
	Nausea(+), vomiting (–), bloody stool (–), fever (–), epistaxis (–)
	Excessive bleeding during periods
	Not taking any vitamins
	No family history of bleeding

Physical Examination

General:	A&O X3
VS:	WNL
HEENT:	conjunctival pallor
GI:	no tenderness, no organomegaly
Extremities:	no clubbing, no cyanosis

Differential Diagnosis:

1. Iron deficiency anemia
2. Pernicious anemia
3. Thallasemia
4. GI malignancy
5. Leukemia

Diagnostic Work-ups:

1. CBC with diff
2. Iron/Ferritin/TIBC
3. Hgb electrophoresis
4. FOBT
5. B12/Folate

CASE NO. 28

Mrs. Kathy Metcalf is a 25-year-old female who has a bruised thigh. This is her third hospital visit in the past three months.

Vital Signs:

T 98.5° F
P 76
R 18
BP 110/75

EXPECTED TASKS

1. Gather the necessary clinical information.
2. Perform a focused and pertinent physical examination.
3. Discuss your diagnostic impressions and differential diagnosis with the patient.
4. Discuss work-ups to be ordered.
5. Complete the patient note after seeing the patient.

Spousal Abuse

(Knocks)

Hi, I'm Dr. _______ and I'm here to examine you today. Do you prefer to be called Mrs. Metcalf or Kathy?

- ☐ 1. So, what brings you in today?
- ☐ 2. When did it happen? How did it happen? *(Note any discrepancy between story and clinical presentation.)*
- ☐ 3. Do you have injuries elsewhere?
- ☐ 4. Are you on any kind of medication right now? *(R/O blood thinners or aspirin.)*
- ☐ 5. What's it like at home?
- ☐ 6. How is your relationship with your husband *(or partner)*?
- ☐ 7. What happens if the two of you disagree?
- ☐ 8. How do you resolve your disagreements?

S.A.F.E. screen for domestic violence

- ☐ 9. Do you feel **S**afe or **S**tressed in relationships?
- ☐ 10. Have you ever been **A**bused or **A**fraid in a relationship?
- ☐ 11. Are your **F**riends and **F**amily aware of your relationship problem?
- ☐ 12. Do you have an **E**mergency plan if needed?

- ☐ 13. Do you have kids?
- ☐ 14. Have they ever been abused?
- ☐ 15. Have you had any illnesses or injuries in the past? Any allergies? Have you ever seen a psychiatrist? Did he prescribe any medication?
- ☐ 16. Are your family members in good health?

☐ 17. What's your job? Do you use any tobacco products? Alcohol? How about recreational drugs?

☐ 18. I will be asking some questions of a sensitive nature that will help me better assess your total health. I can assure you that this will all be kept confidential. Is that okay with you? Are you sexually active? Do you use any contraception? Have you ever had unprotected sex? Do you have sexual partners of the same sex, opposite sex or both? How many partners have you had during the past 12 months?

☐ 19. How would you describe your mood? What do you do for recreation? Do you still like to do them now? Do you sleep well? Do you have trouble concentrating? Have you ever felt you wanted to hurt yourself or somebody? *(R/O Depression.)*

Now, I will do a physical exam. Let me wash my hands first. *(Wash hands.)* Let me put this drape on you so you will feel more comfortable.

☐ 20. I will be testing your muscle strength. Can you raise your thigh/leg/foot up/down against my hand? *(Motor)*

☐ 21. I will be touching parts of your thighs, legs and feet and let me know if you feel them. *(Sensory)*

☐ 22. Now I will be testing your reflexes. *(Patellar & Achilles Reflex)* I will be scratching the sole of your foot. *(Babinski)*

☐ 23. I will be inspecting other parts of your body. *(Look for other injuries.)*

Now let me summarize what we have talked about. You came in because of bruised thigh. Based on the history and the physical examination, I believe that this is spousal abuse, but I want to make sure that the bruises you sustained on your back and thigh are not due to something else; so I am ordering some lab tests to find out. I also would like you to talk with a social worker who may be able to help you. Do you have any questions before I go?

Challenging Questions:

I'm afraid my husband will kill me if he finds out I came here.
I hope he won't take revenge on my kids.
I do not have any insurance. What should I do?
How bad are my injuries?
Are you going to call the police? Please don't!

Spousal Abuse

History:

cc:	bruised thigh
HPI:	25 y/o female c/o bruised right thigh which started after she was hit by her husband. She also complained of pain in certain parts of the leg. No meds taken. Movement does not make the pain worse.
PMH:	(+) physical abuse by husband, no accidents, no hospitalization
FH:	children claimed as healthy with no h/o abuse
SocH:	works as an exotic dancer etoh (+) about 1/2 cup per week cig (+) 2 ppd X 5 yrs. illicit drugs (–)
SexH:	sexually active with husband only; (+) gonorrhea 2 yrs. ago but she and her husband were treated for it.

S: no **A:** yes **F:** no **E:** no

Physical Examination:

Gen:	A&O, appears nervous
VS:	WNL
Extremities:	ROM reduced on right thigh; (–) pain with movement
Skin:	ecchymoses on the right thigh and back
Mental:	Mood is sad but consistent with affect No suicidal or homicidal ideation Energy level unchanged

Differential Diagnosis:

1. Spousal Abuse
2. Bleeding Diathesis
3. Depression
4. Medication induced
5. Leukemia

Diagnostic Work-ups:

1. Patient refused any diagnostic work-up

(If patient does not refuse, order CBC with diff, PT, PTT, Bleeding Time, X-ray of affected extremity, dexamethasone suppression test, refer to social work.)

CASE NO. 29

Ms. Elaine Rogers is a 30-year-old female who came in because of missed periods and abdominal pain.

Vital Signs:

T 98.2° F
P 60
R 15
BP 120/80

EXPECTED TASKS

1. Gather the necessary clinical information.
2. Perform a focused and pertinent physical examination.
3. Discuss your diagnostic impressions and differential diagnosis with the patient.
4. Discuss work-ups to be ordered.
5. Complete the patient note after seeing the patient.

Amenorrhea

(Knocks)

Hi, Ms. Rogers, I'm Dr. _____ and I'm here to examine you today. *(Shakes patient's hand.)* How are you doing?

- ☐ 1. So, what brings you in today?
- ☐ 2. Do you feel nauseated especially in the morning? Any vomiting?
- ☐ 3. Any pain in the pelvic area? Did you take any medication? Did you get relief from it?
- ☐ 4. When was the last day of your most recent menstrual period?
- ☐ 5. Have you noticed any changes in the amount and frequency of the flow?
- ☐ 6. At what age did you start having your periods?
- ☐ 7. Do you have a regular cycle? Every how many days?
- ☐ 8. Have you ever been pregnant? How many times?
- ☐ 9. How many children do you have? Any miscarriages? Any abortions?

I will be asking you some personal questions and I can assure you that everything will be kept confidential. Your answers will give me a more accurate perception of what it is that is bothering you. Is that okay with you?

- ☐ 10. Do you use any kind of contraception?
- ☐ 11. Have you ever had unprotected sex?
- ☐ 12. How many sexual partners have you had during the past 12 months? Are your partners of the same sex, opposite sex or both?
- ☐ 13. Do you have any history of sexually transmitted disease?
- ☐ 14. When was your most recent Pap smear? Do you know the results?

- ☐ 15. Do you feel any pain during sexual intercourse? Do you feel pain when you pee?
- ☐ 16. Do you think you are pregnant? Do you have any fever?
- ☐ 17. Have you been hospitalized before? Any history of accidents or injuries?
- ☐ 18. How's your parents' health? How about your brothers and sisters? Do you have kids? How's their health?
- ☐ 19. What type of job do you do? Are you into any sports? Do you drink alcoholic beverages? Do you smoke? Any use of recreational drugs?

We discussed a lot of information. Now, I will be doing a physical examination but let me wash my hands first. *(Wash hands.)* Would you be more comfortable if I put this drape on your legs? *(Drape patient if she says yes.)*

- ☐ 20. I will be inspecting your thyroid.
- ☐ 21. Can you show me with one finger exactly where the pain is?
- ☐ 22. I will be pressing on your belly and you let me know if it hurts.
- ☐ 23. I will be tapping your belly.
- ☐ 24. Does it hurt anywhere in your belly when I press this? *(Rovsing's sign)*
- ☐ 25. I will be bending and rotating your thigh and let me know if you feel any pain. *(Obturator sign)*
- ☐ 26. Can you lie on your left side? I will be stretching your thigh and let me know if you feel any pain. *(Psoas sign)* I will be inspecting your belly. Now I will be listening to your belly.

I think that's all for now. Now, let me summarize what we have talked about. You told me that you have missed your period and you have abdominal pain. At this point, I am considering the possibility of pregnancy, although, I am also considering other things including ruptured ovarian cyst, hypothyroidism, prolactinoma, and acute appendicitis. I will be ordering some tests and once the results are back, we'll sit down and discuss them. Do you have any questions before I go?

Challenging Questions:

Am I pregnant again?
My partner doesn't want another baby.
If this is appendicitis, am I gonna have an operation?
So there's something wrong with my thyroid.
Should I stop running?
What's a prolactinoma?
What causes a cyst to rupture?

Amenorrhea

History

cc:	amenorrhea
HPI:	– 30 y/o WF with missed period
	– Not under emotional stress
	– Not taking any medication
	– LMP was 4 weeks ago; light flow (2–4 pads per day)
	– Pap smear a year ago was normal
PMH:	no h/o of hospitalization
FH:	father has liver disease; mother had breast tumor
SocH:	lives with a partner and 2 kids; cig (–); etoh occasional, recreational drugs (–).
	Ran a marathon 9 months ago.
SexH:	Sexually active with live-in partner using no kind of contraceptive.
OB/Gyn:	G2P2; menarche at 12.

Physical Examination

General:	A&O, not obese
VS:	WNL
HEENT:	no thyroid enlargements, nodulations or tenderness
Abdomen:	slightly protruberant, N ABS X4 quadrants, N variation between dullness and tympany, no guarding, no organomegaly
Skin:	no hirsutism

Differential Diagnosis:

1. Pregnancy
2. Prolactinoma
3. Ruptured ovarian cyst
4. Hypothyroidism
5. Acute appendicitis

Diagnostic Work-ups:

1. Serum HCG
2. LH/FSH/Prolactin
3. Pelvic exam
4. TSH
5. Abdominal U/S

CASE NO. 30

Mr. Joshua Graves is a 70-year-old male who wanted to see you because he has trouble falling asleep.

Vital Signs:

T 98.1° F
P 88
R 18
BP 130/85

EXPECTED TASKS

1. Gather the necessary clinical information.
2. Perform a focused and pertinent physical examination.
3. Discuss your diagnostic impressions and differential diagnosis with the patient.
4. Discuss work-ups to be ordered.
5. Complete the patient note after seeing the patient.

Depression

(Knocks)

Hi, Mr. Graves, I'm Dr. ______ and I'm here to examine you today. How are you?

- ☐ 1. So, what brings you in today?
- ☐ 2. Do you have any episodes of falling or tripping? Since when? How often?
- ☐ 3. Do you feel dizzy sometimes or do you feel any spinning sensation?
- ☐ 4. Have you ever passed out?
- ☐ 5. When did your tremors start? Any family member with the same kind of tremors?
- ☐ 6. Do you have any trouble getting dressed? How about eating, walking around or going to the bathroom?
- ☐ 7. Who does your shopping? How do you keep up with the daily household chores? Are all your bills up to date?
- ☐ 8. Have you had any illnesses or injuries in the past? Any allergies? Have you ever seen a psychiatrist? Did he prescribe any medication? *(R/O Drug-Induced Parkinson's.)*
- ☐ 9. Are your family members in good health?
- ☐ 10. What's your job? Do you use any tobacco products? Alcohol? How about recreational drugs?
- ☐ 11. I will be asking some questions of a sensitive nature that will help me better assess your total health. I can assure you that this will all be kept confidential. Is that okay with you? Are you sexually active? Do you use any contraception? Have you ever had unprotected sex? Do you have sexual partners of the same sex, opposite sex or both? How many partners have you had during the past 12 months?

☐ 12. How would you describe your mood? What do you do for recreation? Do you still like to do them now? Do you sleep well? Do you have trouble concentrating? Have you ever felt that you want to hurt yourself or somebody? *(R/O Depression.)*

☐ 13. Any weight changes? What bothers you more, a hot or cold temperature? Any changes in your bowel movements? *(R/O Hypothyroidism.)*

☐ 14. Now I will be asking you some question and will ask you to do some things that may challenge your thinking. This is important in making an assessment of your total health.

Where are you now?
What is today's date?
Who am I?
Who was the president before Ronald Reagan?
What did you have for breakfast this morning?
What is 8 plus 7? 25 minus 3?
What do you understand when I say "time is money"?
Have you been seeing things other people don't see?

Now I will be doing a physical exam but let me wash my hands first. *(Wash hands.)*

☐ 15. I will be holding your wrist. Now, can you bend your elbow? Now, try to straighten it. *(Cogwheeling)*

☐ 16. Can you get up from your chair and walk across the room and back? *(Get up and go.)*

☐ 17. Can you pick this object from my hand? *(Tremors decrease during activity.)*

☐ 18. Now I will try to feel your thyroid and let me now if you feel any pain when I do it, OK?

☐ 19. I will be listening to your heart.

Thanks for answering all my questions. Now let me summarize. You told me that you have been having problem falling asleep and that ______. After doing the interview and physical exam, I think we are dealing with major depression here. I am also considering other conditions including Parkinson's Disease, hypothyroidism, anemia and a possible malignancy. I will be ordering some blood tests to make sure we're on the right track. Now, do you have any question before I go?

Challenging Questions:

What is malignancy?
Do you mean I'm going nuts?
I'm no wacko, Doc. Maybe, I should seek a second opinion.
I know this started happening after Pamela's accident. *(Patient starts crying and won't stop.)*
I feel so useless.
You need to give me a strong medication.
What test do you do for depression?
What causes Parkinson's Disease?
Does low blood count cause these kinds of symptoms?

Depression

History:

CC:	difficulty going to sleep
HPI:	70 y/o WM c/o insomnia which started 9 months ago after his wife's accident which left her quadriplegic and wheelchair bound. He has experienced weight loss (10 lbs) and a decrease in appetite. He stopped going to church and refuses to go out with friends because he does not feel like it is worth it. He admits he feels sad most of the time, with feelings of worthlessness. ADL-impaired IADL-impaired
PMH:	had appendectomy while he was in the military
FH:	he was adopted so biological parents are unknown.
SocH:	cig (–), etoh occasional, illicit drugs (–)
SexH:	refuses to answer any question regarding this.

Physical Examination:

Gen:	A&O X3
VS:	WNL except BP 130/85
HEENT:	thyroid is smooth without enlargement or nodulation.
Heart:	no murmurs
Extremities:	no tremors, no cogwheel rigidity
Mental:	mood is sad but consistent with affect No suicidal or homicidal ideation Energy level decreased Judgment and cognition not impaired

Differential Diagnosis:

1. Major Depression
2. Electrolyte imbalance
3. Hypothyroidism
4. Anemia
5. Malignancy

Diagnostic Work-ups:

1. Lytes/Magnesium/Phosphate
2. TSH
3. CBC
4. Cranial CT scan
5. PSA

CASE NO. 31

Mrs. Carrie Ann Kittleberger is a 49-year-old female who has had joint stiffness for the past 4 months. She comes to the office for an assessment.

Vital Signs:

T **98.4° F**
P **68**
R **15**
BP **120/85**

EXPECTED TASKS

1. Gather the necessary clinical information.
2. Perform a focused and pertinent physical examination.
3. Discuss your diagnostic impressions and differential diagnosis with the patient.
4. Discuss work-ups to be ordered.
5. Complete the patient note after seeing the patient.

Joint Pain

(Knocks)

Hi, I'm __________, a medical student. I am here to examine you today before my attending sees you. Is that okay with you? Do you prefer to be called Mrs. Kittleberger or Carrie Ann?

☐ 1. So, what brings you in today?
(Mnemonic: LMNOPQRST)
Location: Can you point with one finger exactly where the pain is?
Medications: Are you taking any medication right now?
Nausea and Vomiting, Weakness? Other symptoms?
Onset: When did this start?
Precipitating Factor: What makes it worse? Does it change with the weather?
Quality: How would you describe the pain?
Radiation/**R**elieving Factors: Does it go anywhere? Does it involve other joints? What makes it go away?
Severity: On a scale of 1–10, where 10 is the most painful, at what level would you rank your pain?
Timing: At what time does it usually occur? How often? How long does it last?

☐ 2. Have you ever been hospitalized? Any accidents or injuries? Allergies? Any similar episodes before?

☐ 3. Are your parents living? How's their health? How about your brothers and sisters? Do you have children? How's their health?

☐ 4. What is your occupation? Do you feel stressed at work? Do you use tobacco products? How about alcohol? Do you take any kind of recreational drugs? Who do you live with?

- ☐ 5. I will be asking some questions of a sensitive nature that will help me better assess your total health. I can assure you that this will all be kept confidential. Is that okay with you? Are you sexually active? Do you use any contraception? Have you ever had unprotected sex? Do you have sexual partners of the same sex, opposite sex or both? How many partners have you had during the past 12 months?
- ☐ 6. Have you had any fever recently? *(R/O septic arthritis.)* How about sore throat? *(R/O rheumatic fever.)*
- ☐ 7. Any history of injury to this area?

Thanks for answering these questions. Now I will be examining some parts of your body but let me wash my hands first. *(Wash hands.)* Let me put this drape on so you'll feel more comfortable. *(Drape patient.)*

- ☐ 8. I will be moving your wrist and your fingers. *(Range of motion.)* I will be pressing on the joints of your fingers and wrist. *(Note any swelling, nodules or deformities.)*
- ☐ 9. Can you put your palms together like this? How about putting the back of your hands together like this. *(Phalen's test)*
- ☐ 10. I will be tapping your wrist. *(Tinel's sign)*
- ☐ 11. Can you make a fist, put the thumb under and close the other fingers over it? Now I will move your fists toward each other. *(R/O de Quervain's tenosynovitis.)*
- ☐ 12. Let's check your reflexes now. *(Do biceps, triceps.)*
- ☐ 13. I will be checking the sensation on your hands. *(Sensory)*
- ☐ 14. Can you open you open your hand while I grab your fingers? *(Motor)*

(Important: When checking joints, always test the other side or do both simultaneously if possible. Also check the joints above and below the affected joint, if applicable.)

Now, let me summarize what you've told me. You said you have pain that affects both your right and left hands, occurring most of the time in the morning, and usually lasting for an hour or more. Considering the history you told me and your physical examination, my initial impression of your condition is rheumatoid arthritis — an inflammation or swelling of the joints of the hands. I am also considering other possibilities including osteoarthritis, septic arthritis, gout and SLE so I am ordering some lab work and x-rays to make sure that we're on the right track. Do you have any questions?

Challenging Questions:

What causes arthritis?
Is it due to my diet?
Am I going to have this for life?
You need to give me something to relieve my pain.
What is SLE? What causes it?
I can't go back to work with this pain.
Is this related to my job?

Joint Pain

History:

cc:	joint pain
HPI:	– 49 y/o female c/o joint stiffness in both hands
	– started 4 mos ago with morning stiffness lasting >30 mins
	– now w/pain 7/10 in pain scale, no fever; (–) h/o of trauma to the area
	– provoked by usage; relieved by heating pads and ibuprofen
	– cig (–), etoh (–), recreational drugs (–)
	– works as a social worker — not stressed
	– sex with husband only

Physical Examination:

Gen:	A&O
VS:	WNL
Extremity:	wrist and fingers ROM not limited.
	Slight swelling in DIP joints B/L
	Phalen's (–), Tinel's (–)
	Biceps and triceps reflexes ++
	Sensory intact
	Motor 5/5 on both upper extrmities

Differential Diagnosis:

1. Rheumatoid arthritis
2. Gout
3. Osteoarthritis
4. SLE
5. Septic arthritis

Diagnostic Work-ups:

1. RF/ESR/ANA
2. X-ray of the hands
3. Synovial fluid analysis and C&S
4. Serum uric acid
5. Anti-Smith, anti-dsDNA

CASE NO. 32

Mr. Dustin Foxworthy is a 21-year-old white male who came in with his mother because of "hearing things."

Vital Signs:

T 98.4
P 90
R 19
BP 135/88

EXPECTED TASKS

1. Gather the necessary clinical information.
2. Perform a focused and pertinent physical examination.
3. Discuss your diagnostic impressions and differential diagnosis with the patient.
4. Discuss work-ups to be ordered.
5. Complete the patient note after seeing the patient.

Schizophrenia

(Knocks)

Hi, I'm Dr. ______ and I'm here to examine you today. How are you both?

- ☐ 1. So, what brings you in today?
- ☐ 2. Have you ever been hospitalized? How about accidents or injuries?
- ☐ 3. Are you taking any medication right now? How about in the past?
- ☐ 4. Now, I'd like to know something about your family's health. Has anyone in your immediate family — parents, brothers, sisters and children — ever had surgery or a specific illness that you can think of?
- ☐ 5. Any family member with problems concentrating or thinking clearly? Depression? Thyroid problems?
- ☐ 6. What is/was your occupation? Any history of tobacco use? How about alcohol? Recreational drugs?
- ☐ 7. Now I will be asking you questions of a sensitive nature but is important in making a good assessment of your condition. Are you married? Are you sexually active?
- ☐ 8. Who do you live with? Do you feel safe at home? Do you have somebody you can turn to when you have problems? *(R/O abuse.)*
- ☐ 9. Do you have any trouble dressing? How about eating, walking around or going to the bathroom? *(ADL)*
- ☐ 10. Who does your shopping? How do you keep up with daily household chores and bills? *(IADL)*
- ☐ 11. How would you describe your mood? Have you noticed any changes in your interests? Do you sleep well? Have you ever had thoughts of hurting yourself or other people? *(R/O depression.)*

☐ 12. Have you noticed any changes in your weight? How's your appetite? Do you feel bothered by hot or cold temperature? *(R/O Hypothyroidism.)*

At this point, I will be asking you some questions that will help give me an idea of your total health.

☐ 13. Where are you right now, Mr. Foxworthy? Do you know today's date? Do you know who you're talking to? *(Orientation)*

☐ 14. What did you have for breakfast this morning? Who was the president of the United States before George Bush Sr.? *(Memory)*

☐ 15. What do you get if you subtract 7 from 100? Subtract seven again from the result? *(Attention/Math)*

☐ 16. Do you ever feel like you are seeing things that other people don't see? Have you ever been told that you have very unrealistic goals for yourself? *(Perception~hallucination, delusion)*

☐ 17. What would you do if you saw a $10 bill on the sidewalk? *(Judgment)*

Now, I am going to do a physical exam but let me wash my hands first. *(Wash hands.)*

☐ 18. I would like to listen to your heart and lungs now.

☐ 19. Can you push your arms/forearms/hands upward against my hand? Now let's do it downward.

☐ 20. I will now check the reflexes in your arms. I will now check the reflexes in your legs.

☐ 21. Can you push your thigh/leg/feet upward against my hand? Now let's do it downward.

☐ 22. Can you get up and walk across the room and back?

Now, Dustin and Mrs. Foxworthy, I would like to summarize what I have noted. You said that ______. My initial impression of your condition is schizophrenia but I am also considering other possibilities including major depression, brain tumor, schizophreniform, and electrolyte imbalance. I am ordering some tests which include some blood tests and a CT scan of the head. Do you have any question before I go?

Challenging Questions:

What is schizophrenia?
What causes it?
I know this is all because of that nasty bitch!
Tumor? Do you mean cancer?
What is schizophreniform?
What is electrolyte imbalance?
Do you think I should bring him to a psychiatrist?
Is this due to drugs?
Is he going to be institutionalized?

Schizophrenia

History:

Information source: patient and mother, seem reliable

cc:	"hearing things"
HPI:	– 21 y/o WM, college student brought in by his mother for "hearing things" – started 8 months ago after breaking up with girlfriend – unusual behavior progressively worsened and patient refuses to go to school – started to threaten neighbors last night which prompted neighbors to call 911
PMH:	h/o appendectomy at 13 y/o. NKDA.
FamH:	unremarkable
SocH:	ceased to go out with anybody since 8 mos ago. cig (–), etoh (–), drugs (–)
SexH:	unknown
ROS:	no fever, no shortness of breath

Physical Examination:

Gen:	A&O X2, uncooperative at times
VS:	WNL except BP 135/88
HEENT:	no eye contact
Lungs:	N breaths sounds, no rales
Heart:	No murmurs
Neuro:	intact CN II-XII; DTR ++, motor 5/5 X4 extremities, sensory intact
MMSE:	mood is sad, inappropriate affect No suicidal but positive for homicidal ideation Remote memory impaired; short term memory intact. Cannot do serial 7s Judgment and cognition impaired

Differential Diagnosis:

1. Schizophrenia
2. Brain tumor
3. Schizophreniform
4. Major depression
5. Electrolyte imbalance

Diagnostic Work-ups:

1. CBC
2. Lytes
3. B12
4. EEG
5. CT scan of the head

CASE NO. 33

Mr. Rudy Merriweather is a 53-year-old African-American male who came in because of abdominal pain.

Vital Signs:

T 100 F
P 100
R 14
BP 132/79

EXPECTED TASKS

1. Gather the necessary clinical information.
2. Perform a focused and pertinent physical examination.
3. Discuss your diagnostic impressions and differential diagnosis with the patient.
4. Discuss work-ups to be ordered.
5. Complete the patient note after seeing the patient.

Right Lower Quadrant Pain

(Knocks)

Hi, I'm Dr. ______ and I'm here to examine you today. Do you prefer to be called Mr. Merriweather or Rudy?

☐ 1. So, what brings you in today?
(Mnemonic: LMNOPQRST)
Location: Can you point with one finger exactly where the pain is?
Medications: Are you taking any medication now?
Nausea and Vomiting, Weakness? Other symptoms?
Onset: When did this start?
Precipitating Factor: What makes it worse?
Quality: How would you describe the pain?
Radiation/**R**elieving Factors: Does it go anywhere? What makes it go away?
Severity: On a scale of 1–10, where 10 is the most painful, at what level would you rank your pain?
Timing: At what time does it usually occur? How often?

☐ 2. Have you ever been hospitalized? Any accidents or injuries? Allergies? Any similar episodes before?

☐ 3. Are your parents living? How's their health? How about your brothers and sisters? Do you have children? How's their health?

☐ 4. What is your occupation? Do you feel stressed at work? Do you use tobacco products? How about alcohol? Do you take any kind of recreational drugs? Who do you live with?

- [ ] 5. I will be asking some questions of a sensitive nature that will help me better assess your total health. I can assure you that this will all be kept confidential. Is that okay with you? Are you sexually active? Do you use any contraception? Have you ever had unprotected sex? Do you have sexual partners of the same sex, opposite sex or both? How many partners have you had during the past 12 months?

Thanks for answering these questions. Now I will be examining some parts of your body but let me wash my hands first. *(Wash hands.)* Let me put this drape on so you'll feel more comfortable. *(Drape patient.)*

- [ ] 6. I will be inspecting your belly.
- [ ] 7. Now I will be listening to your belly.
- [ ] 8. Can you show me with one finger exactly where the pain is?
- [ ] 9. I will be pressing on your belly. *(Watch for inspiratory arrest – Murphy's sign.)*
- [ ] 10. I will be pressing on other areas of your belly and you let me know if it hurts or not.
- [ ] 11. I will be tapping on your belly.
- [ ] 12. Does it hurt anywhere in your belly when I press this? *(Rovsing's sign)*
- [ ] 13. I will be bending and rotating your thigh and let me know if you feel any pain. *(Obturator sign)*
- [ ] 14. Can you lie on your left side? I will be stretching your thigh and let me know if you feel any pain. *(Psoas sign)*

Now let me summarize what you've told me. You said you have abdominal pain located in this area. My initial impression of your condition is acute appendicitis but I am also considering other possibilities including hepatitis, and peptic ulcer disease. I am ordering an ultrasound and some blood tests to make sure that we're on the right track. Do you have any questions?

Challenging Questions:

Isn't appendicitis a disease of young people?
What might have caused this?
What kind of blood test are you ordering?
Am I going to have surgery?
I do not have any insurance.

Right Lower Quadrant Pain

History:

A 53 y/o AAM c/o RLQ pain, colicky in character, that started 6 hours ago. Patient claimed that the pain was non-radiating, and has initially started at the periumbilical area that later localized into the R lower quadrant. Pain not relieved by Maalox. He also had diarrhea a day before this consultation. No other meds taken. Never had hospitalization or operation in the past. He feels slightly nauseated, vomited once and has no appetite for food. No painful urination noted.

Physical Examination:

Gen:	A&O X3, appears in distress.
VS:	T: 100° F P: 100 R: 14 BP: 132/79
Abdomen:	non-distended, normal bowel sounds, no palpable mass or organomegaly, tenderness with guarding in RLQ which is exacerbated by coughing, Rovsings's (+), obturator sign (+), psoas sign (+).

Differential Diagnosis:

1. Acute appendicitis
2. Intestinal Obstruction
3. Viral gastroenteritis
4. Peptic Ulcer Disease
5. Hepatitis

Diagnostic Work-ups:

1. CBC with diff
2. Abdominal Ultrasound
3. Fecal leukocyte
4. AXR
5. serum HAV

CASE NO. 34

Mrs. Blodgett called to voice her concern about her 4-month-old daughter's frequent constipation. The baby's vital signs were taken earlier but the child is not available for physical examination at this time. You are asked to talk to the mother on the phone and get the clinical information while waiting for the baby and the father to come back.

Vital Signs:

T 98.5°
P 95
R 18
BP 125/85

EXPECTED TASKS

1. Gather the necessary clinical information.
2. Perform a focused and pertinent physical examination.
3. Discuss your diagnostic impressions and differential diagnosis with the patient.
4. Discuss work-ups to be ordered.
5. Complete the patient note after seeing the patient.

Pediatric Patient

(Answers phone)

Hi, Mrs. Blodgett, I'm ________, a medical student and I'll be asking questions about your child. How are you today?

- ☐ 1. So I understand that your daughter needs a check-up. Does she have any problem in particular?
- ☐ 2. Are there any changes to her sleeping pattern? Have you noticed any visual problems?
- ☐ 3. Is her hearing okay?
- ☐ 4. Any problems with her mouth or throat?
- ☐ 5. Do you feel any enlargement or any bumps in her neck?
- ☐ 6. Have you noticed any weakness of her arms or legs?
- ☐ 7. Does she have any breathing problems?
- ☐ 8. Any changes in her bowel movements?
- ☐ 9. Any problems with urination?
- ☐ 10. Any abnormal bleeding or discharge?
- ☐ 11. What's it like at home?
- ☐ 12. Is she feeding well? Is she breastfed or formula-fed?
- ☐ 13. How was she delivered?
- ☐ 14. Are her immunizations current?
- ☐ 15. Does she smile when you try to make her smile?
- ☐ 16. Does she roll over now?

- ☐ 17. Does she reach for an object with two hands?
- ☐ 18. Does she put everything to her mouth?
- ☐ 19. Can she sit now?
- ☐ 20. Can she transfer an object from one hand to another?
- ☐ 21. Has she been ill since the last time the doctor saw her? Any allergies?
- ☐ 22. Do you have other kids at home? How's their health? How about you and your husband? How's your health?
- ☐ 23. What type of job do you do? How about your husband? Does anybody at home smoke?

I think that's all for now. Now, let me summarize what we have talked about. Your daughter is basically doing well but the next step is for you to bring your child here and I will perform a physical examination on her and we will go from there.

Pediatric Patient

History

cc:	for routine check-up Source: mother
HPI:	– 4 mo. old female scheduled for routine check-up. – sleeps and eats well, no fever, no cough, no colds, no ill-contacts – has occasional episodes of constipation; normal color and odor of urine – (+) h/o rash in hot weather spontaneously disappearing after several days – delivered vaginally without complications and weighed 7 lbs at birth – mother regularly took prenatal vitamins while pregnant – breastfed since birth; she currently weighs 20 lbs – all immunizations current
Growth & Dev't.:	cooed with (+) head lag at 2 mos. smiles, rolls, grabs things with 2 hands, brings objects to midline at 4 mos.
SocH:	– lives in a house where father smokes – she is a wanted child

Physical Examination:

VS:	WNL
Others:	To follow.

Differential Diagnosis:

1. Routine Check-up
2. Hirschprung's Disease
3. Meckel's Diverticulum
4.
5.

Diagnostic Work-ups:

1. Physical Examination
2.
3.
4.
5.

CASE NO. 35

Mr. Siegfred Wright is a 46-year-old male who came in complaining of excruciating pain on the left side.

Vital Signs:

T 98° F
P 105
R 14
BP 130/85

EXPECTED TASKS

1. Gather the necessary clinical information.
2. Perform a focused and pertinent physical examination.
3. Discuss your diagnostic impressions and differential diagnosis with the patient.
4. Discuss work-ups to be ordered.
5. Complete the patient note after seeing the patient.

Left Flank Pain

(Knocks)

Hi, I'm Dr. and I'm here to examine you today. *(Shakes patient's hand.)* By the way, do you prefer to be called Siegfred or Mr. Wright?

☐ 1. So what brings you in today?
(Mnemonic: LMNOPQRST)
☐ 2. **L**ocation: Can you tell me where the exact area of the pain is?
☐ 3. **M**edications: Have you taken any medications for it?
☐ 4. **N** & V and other symptoms: Do you have nausea? Vomiting? Fever?
☐ 5. **O**nset: When did it start?
☐ 6. **P**recipitating factor: What makes it worse?
☐ 7. **Q**uality: How would you describe the pain?
☐ 8. **R**adiation/**R**elieving Factors: Does it go anywhere? What makes it better?
☐ 9. **S**everity: On a scale of 1–10 where ten is the most painful, where will you rank this pain?
☐ 10. **T**iming: What particular time of the day does the pain occur?
☐ 11. Have you had any accidents or injuries in the past? Any illnesses in the past? How about allergies?
☐ 12. How is your parents' health? How about your brothers and sisters? Do you have kids? How's their health?
☐ 13. What type of job do you do? Any heavy lifting or bending? Is it stressful? Do you drink alcoholic beverages? Do you smoke? Any use of recreational drugs? What type of exercise do you do? How often do you do it?
☐ 14. I will be asking some questions of a sensitive nature that will help me better assess your total health. I can assure you that this will all be kept confidential.

Is that okay with you? Are you sexually active? Do you use any contraception? Have you ever had unprotected sex? Do you have sexual partners of the same sex, opposite sex or both? How many partners have you had during the past 12 months?

Thanks for answering those questions. Now, I will be doing a physical examination but let me wash my hands first. *(Wash hands.)* Would you be more comfortable if I put this drape on your legs? *(Drape patient.)*

☐ 15. I will be listening to your lungs.
☐ 16. I would like you to lie down on your back. I will be palpating your kidneys.
☐ 17. Now, can you sit up. *(Assists patient.)* I will be tapping on your side *(CVA tenderness)* I'll do it on the other side, too. *(If pyelonephritis is highly suspected, just do digital pressure due to extreme pain.)*
☐ 18. I will be checking your belly.
☐ 19. I will be raising your legs. *(straight leg raising test)*

I think that's all for now. Now, let me summarize what we have talked about. You told me that your pain started ______. So, right now my initial impression of your problem is nephrolithiasis or kidney stones. I am also considering other things including a kidney infection, testicular torsion, epididymitis and musculoskeletal sprain. I will be ordering some tests to confirm my diagnosis and we'll go from there. Do you have any questions before I go?

Challenging Questions:

What causes kidney stones?
What causes testicular torsion?
What is epididymitis?
How is this treated?
I've never had this kind of pain before.
I feel like I'm falling apart.

Left Flank Pain

History:

cc:	flank pain
HPI:	46 y/o WM construction worker who came in for sudden, severe L flank pain described as colicky, radiating to the back and the groin area. No meds taken. No history of trauma; no previous similar episode of pain; no h/o hospitalization. No N&V. Denies any blood in urine or stool. No urinary frequency or urgency. Etoh (–), cig (–), illicit drug (–).

Physical Examination:

VS:	WNL except BP 130/85 and HR 105
Gen:	in constant motion and demanding meds for pain relief
Lung:	(+) CVA tenderness on the L side; N BS, symmetrical B/L, no crackles, no dullness, N vocal and tactile fremitus
Abd:	NABS X4 quadrants, no guarding, no tenderness, N variation of dullness and tympany.
Back:	straight leg raising test (–)

Differential Diagnosis:

1. Nephrolithiasis
2. Pyelonephritis
3. Testicular torsion
4. Epididymitis
5. Musculoskeletal sprain

Diagnostic Work-ups:

1. Abdominal X-ray
2. Renal ultrasound
3. CBC/lytes, calcium, phosphate
4. Urinalysis
5. Genital exam

APPENDICES

Institutions Known To Offer Observerships to IMGs

1. Miami Children's Hospital
   Attn: Marco Danon, M.D.
   Department of Medical Education
   3100 S.W. 62nd Ave.
   Miami, Florida 33155

   The observership is contingent on the faculty's availability and are offered in the following fields: Allergy/Immunology, Cardiology, Dermatology, Endocrinology, Gastroenterology, Genetics, Hematology/Oncology, Inpatient Pediatrics, Nephrology, Neurology, Pulmonary Medicine, Radiology, Rheumatology, Pediatric Surgery.

2. University of Miami
   Andrea Ruiz
   Department of Medicine (R-760)
   Office of Academic Affairs
   P. O. Box 016760
   Dominion Towers, 807D
   Miami, Florida 33101
   (305) 243-8273
   (305) 243-5819 Fax

3. Baptist-Lutheran Medical Center
   Medical Student Elective in Family Medicine and Observership for IMGs
   6650 Troost Ave., Suite 305
   Kansas City, MO 64131
   (816) 276-7650
   (816) 276-7090 Fax
   Contact Dr. Jon Welsh at 816-276-7650 or fax 816-276-7090.
   jon.welsh@hcamidwest.com

4. Harvard Medical School
   Department of PM&R at
   Spaulding Rehabilitation Hospital
   125 Nashua St., 5th Floor
   Boston, MA 02114
   (617) 573-7000
   http://spauldingrehab.org/body.cfm?id=265

   Clinical Observership Program is available to international medical students, residents, fellows or physicians (MD/DO) who wish to expand their knowledge of physical medicine and rehabilitation.

5. Mount Sinai Medical Center & Miami Heart Institute
   4701 Meridian Ave.
   Miami Beach, FL 33140
   Mount Sinai, FL offers a paid observership or "mini residency program"
   where you have to pay around $300 per month.

6. D C General Hospital
   1900 Massachusetts Ave. SE
   Washington, DC 20003
   (202) 675-5000

7. Texas Scottish Rite Hospital for Children
   2222 Welborn St.
   Dallas, Texas 75219
   Main Number (214)-559-5000; (800)-421-1121
   tsrh@tsrh.org

   I did an observership in this hospital's Department of Pediatric Orthopedics. It was a great experience and people there were so nice. At the time when I did it, they were providing free lunch and free lodging. Contact them to verify if they still offer the same thing.

8. Maricopa Medical Center
   2601 East Roosevelt St.
   Phoenix, AZ 85008

9. Hahnemann University Hospital
   230 North Broad St.
   Philadelphia, PA 19102

10. Emory University Hospital
    1364 Clefton Rd. NE
    Atlanta, GA 30322

11. Harbor Hospital Center
    3001 S Hanover St.
    Baltimore, MD 21230

12. Providence Hospital
    1150 Varnum St. NE
    Washington, DC 20017

13. Indiana University Medical Center
    550 University Hospital
    Indianapolis, IN 46202

14. Tulane University Hospital
    1415 Tulane Ave
    New Orleans, LA 70112

15. Saint Louis University Hospital
    3635 Vista at Grand Blvd., Box 15250
    Saint Louis, MO 63111

16. University of Kentucky Hospital
    800 Rose St.
    Lexington, KY 40536

17. St. Barnabas Medical Center
    94 Old Short Hills Rd
    Livingston, NJ 07039

18. Fairview Hospital
    18101 Lorain Ave
    Cleveland, OH 44111

19. Oswego Hospital
    110 W. 6th St.
    Oswego, NY 13126

20. KUMC at Wichita
    1010 N. Kansas
    Wichita, KS 67214
    316-293-2600
    kusmw@kumc.edu
    http://wichita.kumc.edu/

21. Baylor College of Medicine-
    Section of International Medicine
    6550 Fannin, Suite 1200
    Houston, TX 77030
    http://www.bcm.edu/medicine/intlmed/intlapp.htm

The following Sections accept International Observers. Contact them by e-mail or telephone to find a sponsoring physician:

Cardiology
Robert Roberts, MD
6550 Fannin, Suite 677
Houston, TX 77030
rroberts@bcm.tmc.edu

Gastroenterology
David Graham, MD
6550 Fannin, Suite 1122
Houston, TX 77030
dgraham@bcm.tmc.edu

Immunology, Allergy, Rheumatology
David P. Huston, MD
One Baylor Plaza, BCM 285, Suite 672E
Houston, TX 77030

Geriatrics
George Taffet, MD
6550 Fannin, Suite 1150
Houston, TX 77030
gtaffet@bcm.tmc.edu

Hematology/Oncology
Garrett Lynch, MD
6550 Fannin, Suite 1057
Houston, TX 77030
lynch@bcm.tmc.edu

Infectious Diseases
David Tweardy, MD
One Baylor Plaza, N-317
Houston, TX 77030
dtweardy@bcm.tmc.edu

Nephrology
Richard Johnson, MD
6550 Fannin, Suite 1287
Houston, TX 77030
rjohnson@bcm.tmc.edu

Pulmonary
1504 Taub Loop, #6PF80002 Pulmonary
Houston, TX 77030
dshelly@bcm.tmc.edu

Thrombosis Research
Paul Bray, MD
One Baylor Plaza, N-317
Houston, TX 77030
pbray@bcm.tmc.edu

If you are interested in an observership in the Michael E. DeBakey Department of Surgery, Baylor College of Medicine, or if you have additional questions about the program, call (713) 798-6078 or send e-mail to: *studentprograms@bcm.tmc.edu*.

22. The Cleveland Clinic Foundation
    9500 Euclid Ave.
    Cleveland, OH 44195
    (216) 444-2200
    (800) 223-2273, ext. 48950
    http://www.clevelandclinic.org/ic/educ/observer.htm

International Physician Observers are physicians selected to visit the Cleveland Clinic for one month to observe procedures in their designated specialty. Applications are competitively reviewed and must be completed and received by June 1st or December 1st for observerships in the following calendar year.

23. Johns Hopkins Hospital
    600 N. Wolfe St.
    Baltimore, MD 21287
    http://www.jhintl.net/JHI/English/Doctors/Observerships_Visits/

Limited to practicing physicians, ideally in early to mid-career. Medical students or physicians who have not yet completed their residency training in a specialty are not eligible to apply.

24. Mayo Clinic offers observership for free at all three Mayo locations. Check their website at *http://www.mayoclinic.org*. Their addresses are printed below:

    Mayo Clinic
    13400 East Shea Blvd.
    Scottsdale, AZ 85259
    (480) 301-8000

    Mayo Clinic
    200 First St. SW
    Rochester, MN 55905
    (507) 284-2511

    Mayo Clinic
    4500 San Pablo Rd.
    Jacksonville, FL 32224
    (904) 953-2000

Additional Hospitals Offering Observerships as Posted in Various Online Forums:

Church Hospital-Baltimore

Meridia Huron Hospital OH

Einstein/Jacobi OH

SUNY (Brooklyn)

University of Rochester, HIV Program

Ann Harbor Hospital, Baltimore

Providence Hospital, Washington DC

VA Hospital, Washington DC

St. John's Hospital and Memorial Medical Center
(Southern Illinois University)

San Joaquin General Hospital in Stockton, California

Stanford University

University of Pittsburg (Department of Critical Care Medicine)

IMG-FRIENDLY HOSPITALS

Legend:
GC — Green Card Holders / US Citizens
H1 — Sponsors H-1B Temporary Worker Visa
J1 — Sponsors J-1 Exchange Visitor Visa

Alabama:
University of South Alabama, Mobile, AL (J1)

Arizona:
University of Arizona, Tucson, AZ (J1)

Arkansas:
University of Arkansas for Medical Sciences, Little Rock, AR (H1, J1)

California:
Alameda County Hospital, Highland, CA
Kern Medical Center, Bakersfield, CA (J1)
St. Mary's Hospital, San Francisco, CA
University of California, Davis, CA (J1)
University of California, San Francisco, CA (J1)
University of Southern California, Los Angeles, CA

Colorado:
University of Colorado Health Sciences Center, Denver, CO (J1)

Connecticut:
Bridgeport Hospital, Bridgeport, CT (GC, H1, J1)
Danbury Hospital, Danbury, CT (GC, H1, J1)
Hospital of St. Raphael, New Haven, CT (GC, H1, J1)
Norwalk Hospital, Norwalk, CT (GC, H1, J1)
St. Vincent's Medical Center, Bridgeport, CT (GC, H1, J1)
University of Connecticut, Farmington, CT (GC, J1)
Yale-New Haven Medical Center, New Haven, CT (J1)

District of Columbia (Washington, DC):
District of Columbia General Hospital, Washington, DC (J1)
Howard University Hospital, Washington, DC (GC, H1, J1)
Providence Hospital, Washington, DC (GC, H1, J1)

Florida:
Mount Sinai Medical Center of Florida, Miami Beach, FL (GC, H1, J1)
University of Florida at Jacksonville, Jacksonville, FL (GC, J1)

Hawaii:
University of Hawaii, Honolulu, HI (J1)

Illinois:
Cook County Hospital, Chicago, IL (GC, H1, J1)
FUHS/Chicago Medical School, Chicago, IL (not disclosed)
Illinois Masonic Medical Center, Chicago, IL (not disclosed)
Jackson Park Hospital, Chicago, IL (GC)
Mercy Hospital, Chicago, IL (GC, J1)
Ravenswood Hospital, Chicago, IL (GC, J1)
Rush Copley Medical Center, Aurora, IL (GC, J1)
Rush Presbyterian Hospital, Chicago, IL (GC, J1)
Rush Westlake, Melrose Park, IL (GC, J1)
St. Francis Hospital, Evanston, IL (GC, H1, J1)
University of Illinois at Urbana-Champaign, Champaign, IL (GC)
University of Illinois at Chicago, Chicago, IL (GC, J1)
University of Illinois/Michael Reese Hospital, Chicago, IL (GC, J1)
University of Illinois at Peoria, Peoria, IL (not disclosed)

Indiana:
Indiana University, Indianapolis, IN (J1)
Ball Memorial Hospital, Muncie, IN (H1, J1)

Kansas:
University of Kansas Medical Center, Kansas City, KS (J1)

Louisiana:
Louisiana State University Health Center, Baton Rouge, LA (J1)

Maryland:
Franklin Square Hospital, Baltimore, MD (GC)
Good Samaritan Hospital, Baltimore, MD (GC, J1)
Harbor Hospital, Baltimore, MD (GC, H1, J1)
Maryland General Hospital, Baltimore, MD (GC, H1, J1)
Prince George's Hospital, Cheverly, MD (GC)
St. Agnes Health Care, Baltimore, MD (GC, J1)

Massachusetts:
Brigham and Women's Hospital, Boston, MA (H1, J1)
Massachusetts General Hospital, Boston, MA (H1, J1)
St. Elizabeth Medical Center of Boston, Boston, MA (J1)

Michigan:
Henry Ford Hospital, Detroit, MI (GC, J1)
Hurley Medical Center/MSU, Flint, MI (GC, J1)
McLaren Regional Medical Center, Flint, MI (GC)
Michigan State University, East Lansing, MI (GC, H1, J1)
Midmichigan Medical Center, Midland, MI (GC)
Providence Hospital, Southfield, MI (GC, J1)
Saginaw Cooperative Hospitals, Saginaw, MI (not disclosed)

St. Joseph's Mercy Hospital, Pontiac, MI (GC, H1, J1)
St. John Hospital, Detroit, MI (GC, J1)
Wayne State University, Detroit, MI (GC, J1)
William Beaumont Hospital, Royal Oak, MI (J1)

Missouri:
St. Mary's Hospital, St. Louis, MO (GC)
St. Lukes Hospital, St. Louis, MO (J1)

Nebraska:
Creighton University/University of Nebraska, Omaha, NE (H1, J1)

New Jersey:
Atlantic City Medical Center, Atlantic City, NJ (GC, J1)
Jersey Shore Medical Center, Neptune, NJ (GC)
Monmouth Medical Center, Long Branch, NJ (GC, J1)
Mountainside Hospital, Montclair, NJ (not disclosed)
Mount Sinai, Englewood, NJ (not disclosed)
Mount Sinai, Jersey City, NJ (GC)
Muhlenberg Regional Medical Center., Plainfield, NJ (GC, J1)
Overlook Hospital, Summit, NJ (GC)
Raritan Bay Medical Center, Perth Amboy, NJ (GC)
St. Barnabas Medical Center, Livingston, NJ (GC)
St. Joseph's Medical Center, Paterson, NJ (GC)
St. Francis Medical Center, Trenton, NJ (not disclosed)
UMDNJ, Pistacaway, NJ (GC)
UMDNJ, Newark, NJ (GC)
UMDNJ, Camden, NJ (GC, J1)
UMDNJ, New Brunswick, NJ (GC, J1)

New Mexico:
University of New Mexico, Albuquerque, NM (J1)

New York:
Albert Einstein/Jacobi Medical Center, Bronx, NY (GC, H1, J1)
Bronx Lebanon Hospital, Bronx, NY (GC)
Brooklyn Hospital, Brooklyn, NY (GC)
Brookdale University Hospital, Brooklyn, NY (GC, H1, J1)
Catholic Medical Center, Jamaica, NY (GC)
Lincoln Medical and Mental Health Center, Bronx, NY (GC)
Maimonides Hospital, Brooklyn, NY (GC, H1, J1)
New York Hospital and Medical Center of Queens/Cornell University, Flushing, NY (GC, H1, J1)
New York Methodist Hospital/Wyckoff Heights, Brooklyn, NY (GC, H1, J1)
NYMedical College (Metropolitan) Hospital, New York, NY (GC, J1)
NYMedical College (Sound Shore) Hospital, New Rochelle, NY (GC, H1, J1)

Our Lady of Mercy Medical Center (offers visa for pre-match), Bronx, NY
St. Barnabas Hospital, Bronx, NY (GC, H1, J1)
St. Lukes Hospital, New York, NY (GC, J1)
St. Joseph's Hospital, Elmira, NY (not disclosed)
St. John's Episcopal South Shore Hospital, Fair Rockaway, NY (GC, H1, J1)
SUNY at Brooklyn, Brooklyn, NY (GC, H1, J1)
SUNY at Buffalo, Buffalo, NY (GC, H1, J1)
SUNY at Syracuse, Syracuse, NY (GC, J1)
Winthrop University Hospital, Mineola, NY (GC, J1)
Woodhull Medical Center, Brooklyn, NY (GC, J1)

Nevada:
University of Nevada, Reno, NV (GC, J1)
University of Nevada, Las Vegas, NV (GC, J1)

North Carolina:
Pitt County Memorial Hospital/East Carolina University, Greenville, NC (J1)
Duke University, Durham, NC (H1, J1)
Wake Forest University School of Medicine, Winston-Salem, NC (J1)

North Dakota:
University of North Dakota, Grand Fork, ND (J1)

Ohio:
Fairview Hospital, Cleveland, OH (GC, J1)
Good Samaritan Hospital, Cincinnati, OH (GC)
Meridia Huron Hospital, East Cleveland, OH (GC, H1, J1)
Mount Sinai of Cleveland, Cleveland, OH (GC)
The Cleveland Clinic, Cleveland, OH (H1, J1)

Oregon:
Oregon Health & Science University, Portland, OR (J1)

Pennsylvania:
Abington Memorial Hospital, Abington, PA (GC, H1, J1)
Allegheny General Hospital, Pittsburgh, PA (GC, J1)
Easton Hospital, Easton, PA (GC)
Frankford Hospital, Philadelphia, PA (H1, J1, GC)
Guthrie Healthcare, Sayre, PA (GC)
Lehigh Valley Hospital, Allentown, PA (GC)
Mercy Catholic Medical Center, Darby, PA (H1, J1)
Mercy Hospital of Pittsburg, Pittsburgh, PA (H1, J1)
MCP Hahnemann University Hospital-Drexel University, Philadelphia, PA (H1, J1)
Montgomery FPR Program, Norristown, PA (H1, J1)
Pinnacle Health/Polyclinic Hospital, Harrisburg, PA (GC)
The Medical Center, Beaver, PA (not disclosed)

University Health Center of Pittsburg, Pittsburg, PA (GC)
UPMC Health System/Shadyside Hospital, Pittsburg, PA (GC)
York Hospital, York, PA (H1, J1)

Rhode Island:
Miriam Hospital of Brown University, Providence, RI (GC, J1)
Roger Williams Hospital, Providence, RI (GC)

South Carolina:
Medical University of South Carolina, Charleston, SC (H1, J1)

Tennessee:
University of Tennessee Medical Center, Knoxville, TN (J1)
Vanderbilt University, Nashville, TN (J1)

Texas:
Texas Tech University, El Paso, TX (GC, J1)
Texas Tech University, Odessa, TX (GC)
Texas Tech University, El Paso, TX (GC, J1)
University of Texas Medical Branch at Galveston, Galveston, TX (H1, J1)

Virginia:
Medical College of Virginia/Commonwealth University, Blackstone, VA (J1)
University of Virginia, Roanoke Salem, VA (GC, J1)

West Virginia:
West Virginia University Hospital, Morgantown, WV (GC, J1)

Washington:
University of Washington, Seattle, WA (J1)

Wisconsin:
Marshfield Clinic-St. Joseph Hospital, Marshfield, WI (H1, J1)
Medical College of Wisconsin, Milwaukee, WI (H1, J1)
Sinai Samaritan Medical Center, Milwaukee, WI (not disclosed)

STATE-SPECIFIC USMLE ATTEMPT LIMITS

Alabama	Three attempts for Step 3. Fourth attempt requires board approval and additional training.
Alaska	Two attempts per step.
Arizona	None.
Arkansas	Six attempts at USMLE Step 3.
California	Unlimited.
Colorado	Unlimited.
Connecticut	Unlimited.
Delaware	Six attempts to pass Step 3.
District of Columbia	Three attempts at USMLE Step 3.
Florida	Five attempts for all steps combined.
Georgia	Three attempts at each step.
Hawaii	Unlimited.
Idaho	Two attempts for each step.
Illinois	Five attempts for all steps combined.
Indiana	Five attempts at each step.
lowa	Six attempts for Steps 1 and 2. Three attempts only for Step 3.
Kansas	Three attempts at Step 3.
Kentucky	Unlimited.
Louisiana	Unlimited for Step l; four attempts at Steps 2 and 3. Fourth attempt at Step 3 requires board approval.
Maine	Unlimited for Steps 1 and 2; three attempts for Step 3. Additional Step 3 attempts require board approval.
Maryland	Four attempts at each step.
Massachusetts	Six attempts at Step 3.
Michigan	Unlimited.
Minnesota	Three attempts at each step.

Mississippi	Unlimited for Steps 1 and 2. Four attempts at Step 3.
Missouri	Three attempts at Step 3.
Montana	Three attempts at Step 3.
Nebraska	Four attempts at each step. One year training for additional attempt on Step 3.
Nevada	Unlimited.
New Hampshire	Three attempts for all steps.
New Jersey	Five attempts at Step 3.
New Mexico	Six attempts at each step.
New York	Unlimited.
North Carolina	Six attempts per step.
North Dakota	Unlimited.
Ohio	Unlimited.
Oklahoma	Three attempts at Step 3.
Oregon	Three attempts at Step 3.
Pennsylvania	Three attempts at Step 3. Additional attempts require board approval after additional training.
Puerto Rico	No information available at time of printing.
Rhode Island	Five attempts at Step 3.
South Carolina	Four attempts at each step.
South Dakota	Three attempts at each step.
Tennessee	Unlimited.
Texas	Three attempts at Step 3.
Utah	Unlimited attempts for Steps 1 and 2. Three attempts for Step 3.
Vermont	Two attempts at Step 3.
Virginia	Unlimited.
Washington	Three attempts at Step 3; one additional attempt with approval (allopathic); unlimited (osteopathic).

West Virginia	Unlimited.
Wisconsin	Three attempts for all steps.
Wyoming	Three attempts at Step 3.

MEDICAL TERMS IN LAYMAN'S LANGUAGE

Alopecia = baldness
Amenorrhea = no period
Anaphylaxis = severe allergy
Aneurysm = bulge in the blood vessel
Angiography = x-ray of the blood vessel
Angioplasty = repair or replace an obstructed blood vessel
Anhedonia = loss of pleasure
Anicteric = no yellowing
Aphasia = can't talk, loss of ability to understand and use language
Apoplexy = stroke
Arthroscopy = use of a viewing instrument to see the joints
Ascites = excess fluid in the belly
Ataxia = unsteady movement
Atherosclerosis = fat deposits in the blood vessels
Barium Swallow = ingesting a dye to enable seeing the internal organs
Breech presentation = feet first or butt first
Bruxism = teeth grinding
Cannabis sativa = marijuana, pot
Carcinoma = cancer
Catatonia = fixed or not moving
Catheterization = putting a tube in
Cauterization = scooping off
Cephalic = head
Cerumen = earwax
Cervix = opening of the uterus
Chancre = painless ulcer in the genitals
Chancroid = painful ulcer in the genitals
Cicatrix = scar
Cirrhosis = scarring of the liver
Cocaine = crack
Colonoscopy = visual exam of the colon
Colostomy = opening from the colon to the surface of the tummy
Colposcopy = insertion of an instrument to see the cervix
Condylomata acuminata = genital warts
Coprolalia = obscene language
Coronary thrombus = blood clot in the blood vessel in the heart
Credits = noise within a joint
Cyanotic = bluish skin
Defecation = poop, bowel movement
Delirium tremens = alcoholic seizure
Delusion = erroneous belief
Dementia = memory loss

Diacetylmorphine = narcotic, heroin
Diaphoretic = excessive sweating
Diarrhea = loose bowel movement, frequent pooping
Dilatation and curettage = removal of tissues from the womb
Dilation and evacuation = removal of tissues from the womb
Dysentery = severe diarrhea due to intestinal infection
Dysmenorrhea = painful period
Dyspareunia = painful sexual intercourse
Dyspepsia = painful digestion
Dyspnea = difficulty breathing
Dysuria = burns when you pee
Ecchymosis = bruise
Eclampsia = high blood pressure in pregnancy causing unconsciousness & convulsions
Ectopic = abnormal location
Ectopic pregnancy = baby located outside the womb
Edema = swelling
Electrocardiogram = instrument that records the electrical activity of the heart
Emesis = vomiting
Endoscopy = insertion of a thin tube to see the inside of the body
Enuresis = bedwetting
Epidural = outer covering of brain or spinal cord, spinal injection to control pain
Episiotomy = cutting an area between the vagina and the anus
Epistaxis = nosebleeds
Eructation = belching/burping
Erythema = redness
Erythroxylon coca = crack, cocaine
Evisceration = removal of contents
Facies = facial appearance
Febrile = with fever
Fetus = unborn baby
Fistula = abnormal connection
Flaccid = limp
Flatulence = excessive gas/farting
Fremitus = vibration
Fugue state = abnormal forgetfulness
Furuncle = infectious, raised lump under the skin
GERD = persistent heartburn
Glossoplegia = heaviness of tongue, paralyzed tongue
Gonad = sex organ in male or female
Gonorrhea = infectious sexually transmitted disease
Halitosis = bad breath
Hansen's disease = leprosy
Hematuria = blood in the urine

Hemorrhage = bleeding
Hepatomegaly = enlarged liver
Hernia = protrusion of an organ outside the body cavity
Heroin = narcotic
Histrionic = attention-seeking personality disorder
Hyperactivity = excessive physical activity
Hyperemesis gravidarum = excessive vomiting during pregnancy
Hyperhidrosis = profuse sweating
Hyperpnea = rapid breathing
Hypertension = high blood pressure
Hypochondria = excessive anxiety over a symptom or ailment
Hypoparathyroidism = low calcium in the blood
Hysterectomy = removal of the womb (uterus)
Ileostomy = opening in the belly where stool can pass out
Inebriated = intoxicated
Insomnia = inability to sleep
Intermittent claudication = pain in the calf muscle during exercise
Interstitial cystitis = painful urination due to swollen bladder
Ischemia = decreased flow of blood
Laparoscopy = insertion of an instrument to see the inside of the body
Lethargy = excessive tiredness
Leukemia = cancer of the blood
Lumbar puncture = needle insertion in the lower back to get brain fluid
Lupus erythematosus = tissue disorder affecting skin, joints & internal organs
Malingering = faking an illness for financial gain
Mastectomy = removal of breast
Mastitis = swollen breasts
Menopausal = period stops
Menorrhagia = excessive bleeding during menstrual periods
Menstruation = period
Methyl amphetamine = speed, illicit drug
Metrorrhagia = abnormal bleeding in between normal periods
Migraine = severe headache
Multiple sclerosis = loss of brain tissue covering
Myalgia = muscle aches
Myocardial infarction = heart attack
Myoclonic seizure = convulsions
Myopathy = muscle disorder
Narcolepsy = excessive sleepiness, uncontrolled sleep pattern
Nasal = nose
Nausea = queasy, urge to vomit, sick to the stomach
Nephritis = kidney inflammation
Nephropathy = kidney disease
Neurofibromatosis = tumors on several nerves

Nevus = mole
Nocturia = excessive peeing during the night
Nulligravida = never been pregnant
Nulliparous = never given birth
Nystagmus = abnormal movement of the eyeballs
Obtundation = decrease or loss of alertness or consciousness
Onychomycosis = fungal infection of the nails
Orgasm = climax
Orthopnea = difficulty breathing while lying on the back
Osteoarthritis = painful joints due to "wear and tear"
Otalgia = ear pain
Otorrhea = ear discharge
Otoscopy = instrument insertion to see the inside of the ear
Pantalgia = pain over the entire body
Paresthesia = numbness or tingling sensation
Paronychia = nail infection
Paroxysm = fit, attack
Patellar reflex = knee jerk
Percutaneous = through the skin
Perineum = area between the anus and the genitals
Pityriasis sicca = dandruff
Pneumaturia = bubbles in urine
Polyuria = excessive peeing
Porphyria = genetic disease causing tummy pain and mental confusion
Postpartum = after birth
Priapism = painful, continuous erection
Productive cough = cough with gunk
Proprioception = awareness of position and location
Prostate gland = part of a male organ
Prostatectomy = removal of the prostate
Pruritus = itchiness
Pseudocyesis = false pregnancy
Ptyalism = excessive salivation
Pulmonary embolism = blod clot in the blood vessel
Quickening = recognition of the baby's movement
Rhinoplasty = plastic surgery of the nose
Rhinorrhea = nasal discharge
Sarcoidosis = disease affecting lymph node, lungs and other body parts
Scleroderma =disease causing thickening of the skin
Scrotum = testicles
Seborrhea = oily skin
Septicemia = presence of bugs or germs in the blood
Sigmoidoscopy = insertion of a thin instrument to see the inside of the body
Sleep apnea = breathing cessation while asleep

Somatization = numerous physical complaints with no underlying problem
Sonogram = ultrasound, instrument using sound waves to see the internal organs
Sphygmomanometer = blood pressure instrument
Splenomegaly = enlargement of the spleen
Sputum = gunk, phlegm
Strabismus = cross-eyes
Stress incontinence = leakage of urine while coughing, laughing, or sneezing
Stupor = sleepy, reduced consciousness or alertness
Syncope = fainting, passing out
Tachycardia = fast heartbeat
Telangiectasis = widened blood vessels, blotchy skin
Tetany = abnormal muscle contraction
Tinea pedis = athlete's foot
Tinnitus = ringing in the ear
Treponema pallidum = syphilis
TURP = surgical removal of prostate tissue
Tussis = cough
Ultrasound = instrument using sound wave to see the internal organs
Umbilical cord = duct connecting the baby to the mother
Urination = peeing
Urticaria = itchy skin, allergy
Uterine = womb
Varicose veins = blood vessels showing on the skin
Vasovagal syncope = loss of consciousness, fainting
Venereal disease = sexually transmitted disease
Venipuncture = blood draw
Vertigo = dizziness, spinning sensation
Vitiligo = white patches on the skin
Vitrectomy = removal of blood from the eye
Xanthelasma = fatty accumulations at the eyelids
Xerosis = dryness
Xerostomia = dry mouth

MEDICAL ABBREVIATIONS USED IN U.S. HOSPITALS

A&O	alert and oriented
A&P	auscultation and percussion
AB	abortion
ABG	arterial blood gases
ACE	angiotensin converting enzyme
ACE-I	angiotensin converting enzyme inhibitor
aCL	anticardiolipin
ACT	activated clotting time
Abd	abdomen
ADC	average daily census
ADD	attention deficit disorder
ADH	antidiuretic hormone
ADHD	attention deficit hyperactivity disorder
ADL	activities of daily living
Adm	admission
Ad lib	as desired
AF	atrial fibrillation
AFB	acid fast bacilli
AFSF	anterior fontanel soft and flat
AFVSS	afebrile, vital signs stable
AGE	appropriate for gestational age
AgNO3	silver nitrate
AIDS	Acquired Immune Deficiency Syndrome
AK	above knee
AKA	above knee amputation
alb	albumin
alk phos	alkaline phosphatase
ALL	acute lymphoblastic leukemia
AM	morning
AMA	against medical advice
amb	ambulatory
AMI	acute myocardial infarction
AML	acute myelogenous leukemia
ANA	antinuclear antibody
ANC	absolute neutrophil count
ANCA	antineutrophil cytoplasmic antibody
anes	anesthesia
angio	angiography
ANLL	acute nonlymphocytic leukemia
Ant	antibiotics
Anti-SMA	anti-smooth muscle antibody

Anti-dsDNA	anti-double stranded DNA
AP	anteroposterior
APAS	at pleasure; as desired
APS	antiphospholipid syndrome
appt	appointment
APTT	activated plasma thromboplastin time
AR	aortic regurgitation
ARC	AIDS related complex
ARDS	acute respiratory distress syndrome
ARF	acute renal failure
AROM	active range of motion
AROM	artificial rupture of membranes
asa	aspirin (acetylsalicylic acid)
ASAP	as soon as possible
ASD	atrial septal defect
ASHD	arteriosclerotic heart disease
ASLO	anti-streptolysin O
astol	as tolerated
ATN	acute tubular necrosis
AV	arterioventricular

BAER	brainstem auditory evoked response
BBB	bundle branch block
BC	Blood culture
BCG	Bacillus of Calmette & Guerrin
BE	barium enema
BF	breast feeding
B/G; BG	Blood Glucose
BIB	brought in by
bid	two times a day (bis in die)
bilat,B/L, BL	bilateral
BILI	bilirubin
BK	below the knee
BKA	below the knee amputation
BM	bowel movement
BMR	basal metabolic rate
BOW	bag of waters
BP	blood pressure
BPH	benign prostatic hypertrophy
BRP	bathroom privileges
Bs	blood sugar
BS	breath sounds
BSO	bilateral salpingo-oophorectomy
BST	breast stimulation test

BSW	Bachelor of Social Work
BUN	blood urea nitrogen
baso	basophil
BTL	bilateral tubal ligation
BW	body weight
bx	biopsy
C/O, c/o	complaints of, complaining of
C/S	cesarean section
C&S	culture and sensitivity
C	centigrade
C spine	cervical spine
CA	carcinoma
CABG	coronary artery bypass graft
CAD	coronary artery disease
Ca	calcium
Cal	calorie
Cap	capsule
Cat	cataract
cath	catheter
cauc	Caucasian
CBC	complete blood count
cc	cubic centimeters
CC	chief complaint
CCE	clubbing, cyanosis or edema
CCU	Coronary Care Unit
CEA	carcinoembryonic antigen
CEO	Chief Executive Officer
CFO	Chief Financial Officer
CHF	congestive heart failure
chol	cholesterol
Cl	chloride
Cl liq	clear liquids
cm	centimeter
CMV	cytomegalovirus
CNA	Certified Nurse's Assistant
CNS	central nervous system
CO_2	carbon dioxide
cont	continued
COO	Chief Operating Officer
COPD	chronic obstructive pulmonary disease
COS	Chief of Staff
CPD	cephalopelvic disproportion
CPM	continuous passive motion

CPR	cardiopulmonary resuscitation
CRF	chronic renal failure
CRNA	Certified Registered Nurse Anesthetist
CSF	cerebrospinal fluid
CST	contraction stress test
CT	crutch training
CT Scan	computerized axial tomography scan
ctx	contraction
CVA	cerebrovascular accident
CVD	cerebrovascular disease
CVP	central venous pressure
cx	cervix
CXR	chest x-ray
D&C	dilatation and curettage
D&E	dilatation and evacuation
D&S	dilatation and suction
D5W	Dextrose (5%) Water
Dc	discontinue
DDS	Doctor of Dental Surgery
Ddx	differential diagnosis
DIC	disseminated intravascular coagulation
DIP	distal interphalangeal joint
Diff	differential count
DKA	diabetes ketoacidosis
DM	Diabetes mellitus
DOA	dead on arrival
DOB	date of birth
DNR	do not resuscitate
DPT	diptheria, pertussis, tetanus
DUB	dysfunctional uterine bleeding
DVT	deep vein thrombosis
DTR	deep tendon reflex
DTs	delirium tremens
Dx	diagnosis
EBL	Estimated body length
EBV	Epstein-Barr virus
ECG	electrocardiogram
ED	Emergency Department
EDC	Estimated date of conception
EEG	electroencephalogram
EENT	eyes, ears, nose, throat
EFM	external fetal monitor

EGA	Estimated gestational age
EGD	Esophagogastroduodenoscopy
ELF	elective low forceps
EMG	electromyogram
ENG	electronystagmogram
ENT	ears, nose and throat
EOM	extraocular muscles
Eos	eosinophil count
ER	emergency room
ERCP	Endoscopicretrograde cholangipancreatography
ES	electrical stimulation
ESR	erythrocyte sedimentation rate
ETIOL	etiology
ETOH	ethyl alcohol
ETT	endotracheal tube
EVAL	evaluation
exam	examination
ext	external
F/U	follow up
FB	foreign body
FBS	fasting blood sugar
FEVt	timed forced expiratory volume
Fe	iron
FFP	fresh frozen plasma
FH	family history
FHM	fetal heart monitor
FHR	fetal heart rate
FHT	fetal heart tones
fib	fibrillation
FIO_2	fractional inspired oxygen
Flliq	full liquid
FLM	fetal lung maturity
FOB	foot of bed
FS	frozen section
ft	foot
FUO	fever of undetermined origin
FVC	forced vital capacity
FWB	full weight bearing
FWW	front wheel walker
Fx	fracture
G	gravid or gram
GA	gestational age

GB	gallbladder
GBS	Group B Strep
GC	Gonorrhea
GERD	gastroesophageal reflux disease
GFR	glomerular filtration rate
GGT	gamma glutamyl tranpeptidase
GI	gastrointestinal
Gm	gram
GN	glomerulonephritis
GSW	gunshot wound
GT	gait training
gtt	drops
GTT	glucose tolerance test
GU	genitourinary
GVHD	graft-versus-host disease
GYN	gynecology
H/H	hemoglobin/hematocrit
H&H	hemoglobin and hematocrit
H&P	history and physical
HA	headache
HBP	high blood pressure
HCOs	bicarbonate
HCVD	hypertensive cardiovascular disease
Hct	hematocrit
HEENT	head, eyes, ears, nose and throat
Hgb (Hg)	hemoglobin
HIV	human immunodeficiency virus
HL	Heparin Lock
HNP	hemiated nucleus pulposus
HOB	head of bed
HP	hot packs
HPF	high power field (microscopic field)
HPI	history of present illness
HR	heart rate
HAP	Henoch-Schoenlein purpura
HTN	hypertension
HVD	hypertensive vascular disease
Ht	height
Hx	history
H_20	water
H_2O_2	hydrogen peroxide
I&D	incision and drainage

I&O	intake and output
ICU	Intensive Care Unit
IM	intramuscular
INR	International Normalized Ratio
IOL	intraocular lens
IP	interphalangeal
IPPB	intermittent positive pressure breathing
IUD	intrauterine device
IUP	intrauterine pregnancy
IV	intravenous
IV push	intravenous push
IVC	inspiratory vital capacity
1VF	IV fluids
IVP	intravenous pyelogram or IV push
IVPB	intravenous piggyback
in	inch
int	internal
Jt	joint
JVD	jugular venous distention
JVP	jugular venous pressure or pulse
K	potassium
KCI	potassium chloride
KUB	kidney, ureter, bladder
kg	kilogram
KJ	knee jerk
L or l	left
LAO	left anterior oblique
Lab	laboratory
Lap	Laparotomy
lat	lateral
lb	pound
LBBB	left bundle branch block
LCSW	Licensed Clinical Social Worker
LDH	lactic acid dehydrogenase
LE	lower extremity
LFT	Liver function test
LGA	large for gestational age
LLE	left lower extremity
LLH	left lateral heelstick
LLL	left lower lobe (of lung)
LLQ	left lower quadrant

LMH	left medial heelstick
LMP	last menstrual period
LOA	left occipitoanterior position
LOC	loss of consciousness
LOS	length of stay
LOT	left occiput transverse position
LP	lumbar puncture
LR	lactated ringers
LS	lumbosacral
LSD	lysergic acid diethylamide
LUE	left upper extremity
LUL	left upper lobe (of lung)
LUQ	left upper quadrant
LVF	left ventricular function
LVN	Licensed Vocational Nurse
LWBS	left without being seen
Lymphs	lymphocytes
lytes	electrolytes
M.A.E.	moves all extremities
MAEW	moves all extremities well
MAP	mean arterial pressure
MAT	multifocal atrial tachycardia
MCH	mean corpuscular hemoglobin
MCL	mid clavicular line
MCV	mean corpuscular volume
MD	medical doctor
MED/SURG	medical/surgical unit
MEF	maximal expiratory flow
Meds	medicines
Mg	Magnesium
MI	myocardial infarction
MIC	minimum inhibitory concentration
min	minute
MMSE	mini mental status exam
Mod	moderate
MRI	magnetic resonance imaging
MRSA	methicillin-resistant Staphylococcus aureus
MVA	motor vehicle accident
MVP	mitral valve prolapse
N&V	nausea and vomiting

Na	sodium
NA	Nursing Assistant
N/A	not applicable
NAD	no acute distress
NaCL	sodium chloride
NaHCO3	sodium bicarbonate
NB	newborn
neg	negative
neuro	neurological
NG	nasogastric
NH3	ammonia
NKA	no known allergies
NKDA	no known drug allergies
nl	normal
NN	nerves
NP	non-productive
NPO	nothing by mouth
NS	normal saline
NSAID	nonsteroidal anti-inflammatory drugs
NSR	normal sinus rhythm
NST	non-stress test
NSY	nursery
NT	non-tender
NTG	nitroglycerin
N/V/D	nausea, vomiting, diarrhea
NWB	no weight bearing
O_2	oxygen
OA	occiput anterior
OB	obstetrics
OBS	organic brain syndrome
occ	occasional
OCT	oxytocin challenge test
OD	right eye
OK	okay
OM	otitis media
OOB	out of bed
OP	outpatient
ophth	ophthalmology
OR	operating room
ORIF	open reduction, internal fixation
ortho	orthopedic
OS	left eye

OU	both eyes (oculi unitas)
oz	ounce
P&PD	percussion and postural drainage
PA & lat	posterior anterior and lateral chest x-ray
PA	Physician Assistant
PAC	premature atrial contraction
PACU	Post Anesthesia Care Unit
PAT	paroxysmal atrial tachycardia
Pap	Papanicolaou smear test
Para	parity
path	pathology, pathologist
PBI	protein bound iodine
pc	after meals
PCA	patient controlled analgesia
PCO_2	carbon dioxide pressure
PCT	pleural chest tube
PDA	patent ductus arteriosus
PDR	Physician's Desk Reference
PE	physical examination
PEEP	positive end-expiratory pressure
PERRLA	pupils equal round reactive to light and accomodation
Ped/Peds	pediatric
PEG	percutaneous endoscopic gastrostomy
PF	peak flow
PFT	pulmonary function tests
PID	pelvic inflammatory disease
PIP	proximal interphalangeal (joint)
PIT	pitocin
PKU	phenylketonuria
PM	afternoon, evening
PMD	private medical doctor
PMH	past medical history
PMI	point of maximum impulse
PMR	polymyalgia rheumatica
PMS	premenstrual syndrome
PND	paroxysmal nocturnal dyspnea
PO_2	oxygen partial pressure
P04	phosphate
POD	postoperative day
POS	positive
PP	post partum
PPD	purified protein derivative
PRBC	packed red blood cells

PRBOW	prolonged ruptured bag of waters
PROM	premature rupture of membranes
PT	prothrombin time, Physical Therapy
PTA	prior to admission
PTT	partial thromboplastin time
PUD	peptic ulcer disease
PUW	pick-up walker
PVC	premature ventricular contraction
PWB	partial weight bearing
pH	hydrogen iron concentration
Pneumo	pneumothorax
po	by mouth (per os)
post	posterior
postop	postoperative
pre	before
preop	preoperative
prep	preparation
prn	whenever necessary
pt	patient
PUD	peptic ulcer disease
PVC	premature ventricular contraction
q	every (quaque)
q2h	every two hours
q am	every morning
qd	every day
q hs	every night at bedtime
qid	four times a day (quater in die)
QNS	quantity not sufficient
qod	every other day
QS	quantity sufficient
QUAD	quadrant
R/O	rule out
(R)	rectal temperature
R	Right
®	Right
RA	rheumatoid arthritis
RBBB	right bundle branch block
RBC	red blood cells
RBOW	ruptured bag of waters
RBS	random blood sugar
RDS	respiratory distress syndrome
RHD	rheumatic heart disease

Rh	Rhesus blood factor
RL	ringers lactate
RLE	right lower extremity
RLL	right lower lobe (of lung)
RLQ	right lower quadrant
RN	Registered Nurse
ROA	right occiput anterior
ROM	Range of Motion
ROP	right occiput posterior
ROS	review of systems
ROT	right occiput transverse
RR	respiratory rate
rrr	regular rate and rhythm
RSV	respiratory syncytial virus
R/T	related to
RTC	return to clinic
RUE	right upper extremity
RUL	right upper lobe (of lung)
RUQ	right upper quadrant
RV	right ventricle
Rx	prescription
reg	regular
rehab	rehabilitation
sat	saturate
SBO	small bowel obstruction
Schiz	Schizophrenia
sed rate/ESR	erythrocyte sedimentation rate
SFP	superficial femoral artery
SGA	small for gestational age
SGOT	serum glutamic-oxaloacetic transaminase
SGPT	serum glutamic pyruvic transaminase
SH/SocH	social history
SIADH	Syndrome of Inappropriate Antidiuretic Hormone Secretion
SL	sublingual
SLR	straight leg raising
SNF	Skilled Nursing Facility
SOAP	subjective, objective, assessment, plan
SOB	shortness of breath
sol	solution
S/P	status post
Spec	specimen
SPgr	specific gravity
SQ/subq	subcutaneous

SR	sinus rhythm
SROM	spontaneous rupture of membranes
SS#	social security number
S/S	signs and symptoms
Staph	Staphylococcus (bacteria)
STAT	at once (statim)
Strep	Streptococcus (bacteria)
STV	short term variability
SVC	superior vena cava
SVT	supraventricular tachycardia
Subling (SL)	sublingually; under the tongue
Surg	surgery or surgical
Sx	symptoms
T	temperature
T&A	tonsillectomy and adenoidectomy
T&C	type and crossmatch
T spine	thoracic spine
T.U.R.	transurethral resection
tab	tablet
TAH	total abdominal hysterectomy
TB	tuberculosis
tbsp	tablespoon
TEA	thromboendarterectomy
TENS	Transcutaneous Electrical Nerve Stimulator
TIA	Transient Ischemic Attack
tid	three times a day (ter in die)
TKO	to keep open
TLC	total lung capacity
TMJ	temporomandibular joint
TMs	tympanic membranes
TO	telephone order
TORCH	toxoplasmosis, syphilis, rubella, cytomegalovirus, herpes
TPN	total parenteral nutrition
TPR	temperature, pulse and respiration
trans	transfer
tsp	teaspoon
TURBT	transurethral resection of bladder tumor
TURP	transurethral resection of the prostate
TVH	total vaginal hysterectomy
Tx	treatment
U/C	uterine contraction
UA	urinalysis

UE	upper extremity
UGI	upper gastrointestinal
UO	urinary output
URI	upper respiratory infection
US	ultrasound
UTI	urinary tract infection
VA	visual acuity
VBAC	vaginal birth after cesarean
VC	vital capacity
VD	venereal disease
VDRL	venereal disease research laboratories (lab test for syphilis)
VE	vaginal exam
Vent	mechanical ventilator
VO	verbal order, voice order
VRE	Vancomycin Resistant Enterococci
VS	vital signs
VSD	ventral septal defect
VSS	vital signs stable
v, vs	versus
via	by
vol	volume
WBAT	weight bearing as tolerated
WBC	white blood cells
WDWN	well developed, well nourished
WF	white female
WM	white male
WNL	within normal limits
WP	whirlpool
W/U	work up
w/a	while awake
w/c	wheelchair
w/o	without
wk	week
wt	weight
Y/O, y/o	year old
yr	year

STEP 2 CS PATIENT NOTES

History:

Physical Examination:

Differential Diagnosis:

1.
2.
3.
4.
5.

Diagnostic Work-ups:

1.
2.
3.
4.
5.

(photocopy this page to be used for the mock patient encounters)

INDEX

S

T

U

V

W

Made in the USA
Monee, IL
05 November 2026

67853046R00153